Juicing For Life

Cherie Calbom
Maureen Keane

AVERY
a member of Penguin Putnam Inc.

Published by the Penguin Group
Penguin Group (USA) Inc., 375 Hudson Street, New York, New York 10014, USA • Penguin Group
(Canada), 90 Eglinton Avenue East, Suite 700, Toronto, Ontario M4P 2Y3, Canada (a division of Pearson
Penguin Canada Inc.) • Penguin Books Ltd, 80 Strand, London WC2R 0RL, England • Penguin Ireland,
25 St Stephen's Green, Dublin 2, Ireland (a division of Penguin Books Ltd) • Penguin Group (Australia),
250 Camberwell Road, Camberwell, Victoria 3124, Australia (a division of Pearson Australia Group Pty
Ltd) • Penguin Books India Pvt Ltd, 11 Community Centre, Panchsheel Park, New Delhi–110 017, India •
Penguin Group (NZ), 67 Apollo Drive, Mairangi Bay, Auckland 1311, New Zealand (a division of
Pearson New Zealand Ltd) • Penguin Books (South Africa) (Pty) Ltd, 24 Sturdee Avenue, Rosebank,
Johannesburg 2196, South Africa

Penguin Books Ltd, Registered Offices: 80 Strand, London WC2R 0RL, England

Most Avery books are available at special quantity discounts for bulk purchase for sales promotions, pre-
miums, fund-raising, and educational needs. Special books or book excerpts also can be created to fit
specific needs. For details, write Penguin Group (USA) Inc. Special Markets, 375 Hudson Street, New
York, NY 10014.

Library of Congress Cataloging-in-Publication Data

Calbom, Cherie.
    Juicing for life : a guide to the health benefits of fresh fruit and vegetable
juicing / Cherie Calbom, Maureen Keane.
        p.   cm.
    Includes bibliographical references.
    ISBN 0-89529-512-1
    1. Fruit juices—Health aspects. 2. Vegetable juices—Health aspects.
I. Keane, Maureen. II. Title.
RA784.C23   1992   91-39423 CIP
613.2'6—dc20

Printed in the United States of America
66   65   64   63

Neither the publisher nor the authors are engaged in rendering professional advice or services to the
individual reader. The ideas, procedures, and suggestions in this book are not intended as a substitute
for consulting with a physician. All matters regarding health require medical supervision. Neither the
authors nor the publisher shall be liable or responsible for any loss, injury, or damage allegedly arising
from any information or suggestion in this book. The opinions expressed in this book represent the personal views of the authors and not of the publisher.

The recipes in this book are to be followed exactly as written. The publisher is not responsible for specific
health or allergy concerns that may require medical supervision. The publisher is not responsible for any
adverse reactions to the recipes in this book.

While the author has made every effort to provide accurate telephone numbers and Internet addresses at
the time of publication, neither the publisher nor the authors assume any responsibility for errors, or for
changes that occur after publication. Further, the publisher does not have any control over and does not
assume any responsibility for author or third-party websites or their content.

Contents

PART THREE / THE DIET PLANS

Foreword

The Surgeon General's 1989 Report, the Secretary of Health and Human Services, Health America 2000, the National Cancer Institute, and Dietary Goals for the United States all say the same thing: Eat more fresh fruits and vegetables. The problem is that people just don't.

It is now recognized that orange-red vegetables have high levels of carotene, a suspected anticancer substance; that citrus fruits contain vitamin C and bioflavonoids, important immune-strengthening nutrients; and that dark green leafy vegetables are rich in folic acid, a B-complex vitamin necessary for proper maintenance of red blood cells and the nervous system. Unfortunately, people do not generally eat the four to five portions of these fruits and vegetables recommended by the government public health agencies, the medical and nutrition professionals, and the community health activists. Health benefits can be realized only if people eat these important foods.

In *Juicing for Life*, Cherie Calbom and Maureen Keane present juicing as an easy, convenient, and fun way of putting a diversity of flavorful, nutrient-packed beverages into the diet, making good nutrition accessible even to people who think they dislike fruits and vegetables. First, the authors explain the role of juicing in a well-balanced diet plan. Information is then provided on both the preventive and the therapeutic benefits of certain juices. Finally, dozens of juicing recipes are included, demonstarting the many ways in which we can reap the health benefits of various fruits and vegetables. Throughout the book, the emphasis in on fresh produce and and the unrefined diet. This is consistent with contemporary nutritional science, which indicates that the less food is processed, the more food retains its active nutrients.

I found the recipes and juicing suggestions in the book to be very helpful, and feel sure that *Juicing for Life* will open the door to improved nutrition for you and your family.

Jeffrey Bland, Ph.D.
Nutritional Biochemist
Author of
Your Health Under Siege: Using Nutrition to Fight Back

Introduction

Writing about nutrition and juice is my passion. I am convinced that dietary changes—and, in particular, the consumption of large amounts of fresh fruit and vegetable juices—have saved my life. This is why.

I can't remember ever being really healthy and energetic, even as a child. In fact, I remember my grandmother telling me that I was sickly most of the time. I'm convinced my problems began before I was born. My grandmother said my mother had been sickly all her life, too. She died of cancer when I was six years old. As a child, I caught every cold that came along. I missed school often and always had to watch what I did so I wouldn't get sick. I remember going on a hike with a friend at about age twelve and feeling as though I was going to faint because I was so out of breath.

What was surprising was that no doctor ever figured out why I was so tired and why I was always getting sick. Once a doctor thought I had a milk allergy, and when I stopped eating dairy products, I did improve. But that was the extent of the medical help. Not one health professional ever asked my grandmother what I was eating. And what I was eating would probably have killed a strong, healthy gorilla! I can't remember ever eating green vegetables in the winter. Summers offered an abundance of fresh vegetables from Grandma's garden, which I liked. But that was about the only light in the dim tunnel of my diet. The rest of the time I existed on candy bars, potato chips, cookies, sweet rolls, homemade white bread, cake, and potato soup. I did like potatoes. I didn't like any other vegetables, so my grandmother didn't serve them. She almost never cooked any kind of animal protein but eggs. So my diet was supplemented with junk.

When I was fourteen, I went to live with my aunt and uncle, and I remained with them throughout high school and my first year of college. My diet improved in their home, and so did my health. But my weight soared. By that time, I was truly addicted to sweets and ate more than my share, along with all the other foods provided in abundance. Finally, I couldn't stand being overweight, so I went on a starvation diet. I refused meals and snacked on cookies. I lost weight, and six months later almost died of pneumonia.

In my late teens, I discovered the wonders of vitamin and mineral pills and noticed a boost in my energy. But I still ate large quantities of sweets and rejected most vegetables. All through my twenties, I skated the line between sickness and health. My diet had improved somewhat and so had my energy. But I continued to eat too much of the wrong stuff, and I still caught lots of colds and viruses. I was so tired in the morning that I could barely crawl out of bed. Sometimes I felt I'd never make it through the workday because I was so fatigued.

The real turn for the worse came around the time I turned thirty. I had developed a full-blown case of chronic fatigue syndrome that caused me to feel as though I had the flu most of the time. A low back pain kept getting worse. I was diagnosed with hypoglycemia, and later with *Candida albicans* (a systemic yeast infection). And it seemed I had PMS thirty days out of the month! Finally, I went to a holistic medical doctor for allergy testing and walked out with a list of food allergies longer than my grocery list.

I was so sick and fatigued, I finally decided to quit my job. I knew I had to do something quickly because I needed to work again. I was so sick and so tired of being sick that I was ready for any new approach. So I started looking through the books at health food stores and picked up several books that talked about a relationship between diet and health. Then I read Dr. Norman Walker's book about juicing fresh fruits and vegetables.

With nothing to lose but ill health, I bought a juicer, put my furniture in storage, and moved to my family's home for the summer. I first went on the five-day juice fast, drinking mostly vegetable juices and some fruit juices and eating no solid food. I followed the cleansing instructions by taking enemas every day to help eliminate toxins.

For the duration of the summer, I followed a detoxification diet along with periodic juice fasts. By September, my symptoms were virtually gone. I had no more back pain, fatigue, or PMS. Many of my food allergies had disappeared as well. I felt like a new person. I had to follow the anti-Candida program to get rid of my yeast condition, but eventually that was gone too. I'm convinced that those dietary changes saved my life.

There's a lot of talk today about genetic inheritance of disease. But in my research on cancer, I learned that only 2 percent of all cancers are attributable to genetic factors, while 35 percent of all cancers are diet-related, according to the National Cancer Institute. What I had inherited from my mother was her dietary patterns—a love of sweets and a distaste for vegetables and whole grains.

I often ask myself where I'd be today if I hadn't changed my diet. I'll never know for sure, but I think I'd be following in my mother's footsteps. And if that were true, right now I'd have cancer and about six months to live. Instead, at forty-three, I've never felt better. I have more energy than I did when I was twelve. In fact, I can't imagine tiring out on a hike now. I'm not even winded after an hour-and-a-half aerobic workout! In the past two years, I've had enough energy to get a master's degree in nutrition while working part-time at a medical center and writing two books. But that's not all that's changed. I never have to go on a weight-loss diet, because my weight rarely fluctuates more than five pounds. Constantly, people guess my age to be about thirty-something. And best of all, I feel happy to be alive every day.

WHY JUICE?

The juice of fresh fruits and vegetables is the richest available food source of vitamins, minerals, and enzymes. Usually, you just can't eat enough raw fruits and vegetables in a day to nourish your body properly. While this has probably always been true, it is especially true today, when you need extra nutrients to help your body detoxify a large amount of environmental toxins. On most days, you probably can't find the time to eat five pounds of carrots. But you certainly can find the time to drink their nutritional equivalent in a delicious, nutrient-rich glass of juice. That's why juicing is such an important addition to a busy lifestyle!

Juice enables your body to easily assimilate the many valuable nutrients found in food. Enzymes are organic catalysts that increase the rate at which foods are broken down and absorbed by the body. Found in plant foods such as fruits and vegetables, enzymes are destroyed when these foods are cooked. This is why fresh raw produce should constitute at least half of your diet. The quick and easy digestion of these foods, made possible by the enzymes, will give you greater energy and health.

The Juiceman, Jay Kordich, is known for his statement: "All life on earth emanates from the green of the plant." Raw fruits and vegetables are nature's way of giving us life. The late Dr. Bircher-Benner, who founded the famous Bircher-Benner clinic in Europe, said that nothing more therapeutic exists on Earth than green juices. Juice offers you a concentration of nutrients packaged in the best proportions so that you can benefit from the synergistic effect of all nutrients working together to nourish your body and enhance your health. In fact, once your begin drinking juices on a regular basis, you may not need vitamin and mineral supplements. I like to call these drinks "vitamin and mineral cocktails"!

Juicing for Life was designed to help you and your family achieve the greatest health possible. In Part One, you will learn about the nutrients that make up a truly healthful diet, and why juice is one of the best sources of these nutrients. Part Two examines a number of common disorders from acne to water retention, explaining each disorder, offering dietary suggestions, detailing the nutrients that are known to be most helpful for that condition, and listing the juices that can support you during the healing process. Finally, in Part Three, you will find some special diets that will aid you in losing excess weight, in identifying food allergies, in cleansing your body of toxins, and in treating a number of other problems.

Sickness or health—the choice is yours. The physical condition you have tomorrow starts with what you do for your body today. It's up to you! I encourage you to choose vibrant health. Eat fiber-rich foods like fruit and vegetable salads, whole grains, and legume dishes made with beans, lentils, or split peas. Drink two to four glasses of fresh juice daily. Reduce your intake of animal products. Reduce—or, better yet, eliminate—your consumption of junk foods, sweet treats, and refined foods. And don't give up on eating healthfully even if you don't get immediate results. Trust me. You can and will feel healthier, with more energy and greater resistance to disease, when you start juicing for life!

Cherie Calbom
"The Juicewoman"
Nutritionist

PART ONE

The Basics

The Nutrients

G randma used to give great nutritional advice: Eat your vegetables. Over the years, that simple suggestion has been replaced with a lot of complicated-sounding recommendations. Many people end up more confused than enlightened.

Choosing a healthy diet is a lot like putting together a jigsaw puzzle. In the beginning, it's a confusing jumble, but as the pieces fall into place, a picture begins to emerge. The purpose of this book is to help you form your own unique picture of health. Choose a diet from Part Three that suits your particular condition. The result will be a personalized juicing program that will optimize your body's ability to heal itself.

Carbohydrates

The largest piece of our nutrition puzzle belongs to carbohydrates. These macronutrients are the most abundant compounds on Earth, forming the grass under your feet and the trees that fill the sky. They should constitute most of the foods you eat. Carbohydrates are formed when carbon dioxide and water come together in the presence of sunlight and chlorophyll (the pigment that makes plants green). The chemical bonds of the carbohydrate lock in the energy of the sun. This energy is released when the human body burns plant food as fuel.

There are three kinds of carbohydrates:

1. Simple carbohydrates, or sugars, are America's favorite form of carbohydrate. If a food tastes sweet, it's because it contains simple sugars. These quickly absorbed molecules are a ready source of energy for the body. Fruits and some vegetables are good sources of simple carbohydrates. These foods contain a balance of many different sugars, including glucose, fructose, sucrose, and sorbitol. High-sugar manmade foods such as candy bars and soft drinks contain a refined single sugar. Variety, even in your sugar consumption, is prudent. Stay away from refined-sugar foods, and satisfy your sweet tooth with foods that contain both unrefined sugars and other nutrients.

2. Complex carbohydrates, or starches, are your body's best source of energy. Starches are sometimes called polysaccharides (meaning many sugars), because they are composed of strings of simple sugars. Your body slowly breaks down these strings into sugar. This gradual release of sugar keeps the glucose at an even level in the blood, an important fact to remember if you are a diabetic or suffer from hypoglycemia. Starches are your body's best energy source. Good sources of complex carbohydrate are products made with unrefined grains, such as whole grain breads, brown rice, and whole wheat pasta, as well as the root vegetables, such as potatoes and yams.

3. Fiber is the celebrity of the nutrition world. Its importance in the digestive tract has been the object of numerous articles in popular magazines and scholarly journals. Fiber is a type of polysaccharide that resists digestion by your body's enzymes and acids. Soluble fiber forms a gel-like substance in the digestive tract that appears to bind cholesterol so it cannot be reabsorbed. Insoluble fiber is sometimes called nature's broom, because it decreases transit time in your intestine and keeps it swept clean. Fiber is found in fruits, vegetables, unrefined grains, and legumes.

While all types of carbohydrates are important, it is best to eat most of them in the form of polysaccharides. If you have any kind of problem metabolizing sugars—that is, if you have diabetes, a Candida infection, or hypoglycemia—it is best to avoid them altogether.

Fats or Lipids

The next largest puzzle piece belongs to fats or lipids. When animals consume more energy than they can use, the surplus is stored as fat. Fat is a very concentrated source of energy: a gram of sugar brings 4 calories with it; a gram of fat brings 9 calories, more than double that of sugar. Fats are often thought of as being the "bad guys" of the nutrition world, taking the blame for everything from acne to ulcers. But not all fats are created equal. The real "bad guys" are saturated fats. A diet high in saturated fats may increase your risk of developing heart disease and cancer. The "good guys" are vegetable fats such as olive and safflower oil. These oils may decrease your risk of developing heart disease. But the real heroes in this story are the omega-3 fatty acids. This is a type of oil found in cold-water fatty fish such as mackerel, herring, and salmon. Omega-3 fatty acids can decrease the risk of heart attack by making your blood platelets less sticky. They can also reduce inflammation caused by autoimmune diseases such as rheumatoid arthritis. All fats, however, have one thing in common: They cause weight gain when eaten in excess.

Protein

With the addition of protein, our nutrition puzzle begins to take shape. The word protein comes from the Greek word meaning "to take first place." After water, protein is the most plentiful substance in our body; it is an integral part of every living cell. In foods, protein usually comes packaged with fat, and the type of fat determines how "healthy" a protein source is. Red meat contains a lot of saturated fat along with its protein. Fish contains a lot of omega-3 fatty acids. Beans and legumes are excellent low-fat sources of protein when balanced with nuts, seeds, and grains.

Minerals

Our nutrition puzzle would not be complete without minerals. The word mineral means an element in its simple inorganic form. In the body, minerals occur chiefly in their ionic form; metals form positive ions (cations) and nonmetals form negative ions (anions). Minerals can be used for structural tissues, as calcium and magnesium are used in bone, or they may be used in electrolyte balance, as is the case with potassium, sodium, chloride, and calcium. The major minerals are calcium, phosphorus, chloride, magnesium, potassium, sulfur, and sodium. Minerals needed only in tiny amounts are called trace minerals. They include arsenic, chromium, cobalt, copper, fluoride, nickel, selenium, manganese, boron, and vanadium.

Vitamins

The tiniest part of our puzzle belongs to vitamins. Vitamins are substances that are needed by the body for normal growth and tissue maintenance. Even though they are needed in only small amounts, most vitamins must be supplied by the diet because the body cannot manufacture them. They are usually divided into two groups: the water-soluble vitamins and the fat-soluble vitamins. The water-soluble vitamins include the B-complex vitamins and vitamin C. The fat-soluble vitamins include vitamins A, D, E, and K. The body can store the fat-soluble vitamins, but water-soluble vitamins must constantly be replenished. Fruits and vegetables are excellent sources of many vitamins.

Balance

Imagine for a minute that you dropped your "fat" puzzle piece into some water and it swelled, getting much larger. Or maybe the dog chewed on your "carbohydrate" piece, and it shrank. Let's try to put the pieces together. They don't fit, do they? The fat piece is crowding out the protein and minerals. The reduced carbohydrate piece is making the vitamin piece loose.

If you want your body to be fit, your nutrient pieces must fit. That is the problem with the Standard American Diet (SAD): It is out of balance. Every piece is equally important, but only in its proper proportion.

Nutrition Gets Radical

Although free radicals may sound like members of a sixties' political group, they actually represent one of the most exciting discoveries in nutrition today. Free radicals are small molecules with an extra electron. They hurtle through tissue looking for electrons to steal. This shooting spree wounds cell membranes and can damage the DNA codes within the cell's nucleus. When an electron has been liberated, the molecule it leaves is transformed into another free radical, causing even more wounded cells. A chain reaction results. Free radical damage has been implicated in heart disease, cancer, aging, inflammatory problems, Parkinson's disease, periodontal disease, and cataracts. The list is constantly growing longer.

Where do free radicals come from? Some can be generated from air pollution, ultraviolet light, tobacco smoke, some medications, and even some normal bodily functions. Since these "wild bullets" are literally surrounding you, how can you protect yourself from them? Easy. Mother Nature has given us a group of compounds called antioxidants. Like a bulletproof vest, antioxidants protect your cells by scavenging free radicals, binding to them, and carrying them out of your body. Antioxidants can be minerals, vitamins, enzymes, or "anutrient" compounds. The best-known antioxidants are vitamin C, vitamin E, selenium, and beta-carotene.

The Missing Piece: Anutrients

Carbohydrates, fats, proteins, vitamins, and minerals—our nutrition puzzle seems complete. But something is missing; the parts don't quite fit. Shake the frame, and the pieces are loose. What have we lost? Researchers have been asking themselves that question for a long time, and they are finally getting close to the answer. Recently, some investigators suggested the name "anutrients" for those compounds that protect the body from the environment. These compounds have no known deficiency symptoms and seldom produce toxic effects. Anutrients are found in fruits, vegetables, and grains. Some anutrients are pigments such as the carotenes (yellow-red), the chlorophylls (green), the anthocyanins (red-blue), the proanthocyanidins (colorless), and the flavonoids (colorless or yellow). Sulfur compounds, which give the cabbage family its distinctive odor, are also anutrients. The list grows longer every year. It may take decades to identify all the nutrient compounds and even longer to figure out how they work. But don't wait for all the cataloging to be done before you reap the benefits that anutrients have to offer. Your puzzle pieces may start to get loose. Act today. Follow your grandmother's advice: Eat (and drink) your vegetables.

The Benefits of Juicing

According to the American Cancer Society, the National Cancer Institute, and the National Research Council, Americans do not eat enough fresh fruits and vegetables to prevent disease. Yet these are the foods that have powerful protective effects for the body. These protective components have already been explained in the previous section. Now the question to answer is, "How much should we be eating?"

Eat Your Fruits and Vegetables

Many health professionals say that we should eat seven servings of vegetables and two servings of fruits per day. Others say we need even more—that between 50 and 75 percent of our diet should be raw food if we are to enjoy optimal health and abundant energy. Leslie and Susannah Kenton, authors of the book *Raw Energy*, state that a "vast quantity of evidence . . . exists showing that the high-raw diet—a way of eating in which 75 percent of your foods are taken raw—cannot only reverse the bodily degeneration which accompanies long-term illness, but retard the rate at which you age, bring you seemingly boundless energy and even make you feel better emotionally."

Ann Wigmore, founder of the Hippocrates Health Institute, is one of the best advertisements for the raw food diet. Now in her eighties and looking vibrantly healthy and much younger than her years, she teaches people how to recover from illness and maintain vibrant health with "live foods." Ann eats a virtually raw food diet and says it was this diet that helped her recover from illness and chronic fatigue, as well as slow the aging process. She reports that a short time after beginning her raw food diet at the age of fifty, her illnesses disappeared, her energy improved, her gray hair turned dark, and her sagging skin tightened as though she'd had a face lift. Now she teaches thousands of other people how to find the same rejuvenation through live foods.

The late Dr. Max Bircher-Benner, M.D., of the famous Bircher-Benner clinic in Europe, believed that cooking and processing food destroys its living energy. He said that the most nutritive energy is obtained from plants. Plants derive their energy from the sun during photosynthesis, and eating the plants passes this special energy into our bodies. Plants also give the body the "spark plugs" of life: enzymes, vitamins, and minerals. Do you know where enzymes, vitamins, and minerals come from? Minerals are basic constituents of the Earth's crust, and plants "drink them up" from the soil. Enzymes and vitamins are produced in plant tissues. When we consume live food, we bathe the trillions of cells in our bodies with these plant-derived nutrients.

If you want to be healthier, recover from illness, have more energy, and slow the aging process, eat more fresh, raw vegetables and fruit. And get rid of the junk food! When you indulge in culinary excesses, detoxify your body with a cleansing diet. (See the Cleansing Diets on page 299.) Make healthful eating a way of life.

Why Do We Need Juice?

Unless you are already eating three-quarters of your diet raw, we suggest you eat more raw foods. We know that on most days, if you're like the average American, you don't come close to getting even two bowls of raw food. One recent study revealed that most Americans eat no more than one to three salads a week. So here's the crucial question: How are you going to make every meal at least one-half to three-quarters raw food? Sit down and plan out a day. Plan out a week. Can you manage this high raw-food regimen every meal of every day? If you're like the nutrition patients of one of this book's authors, Cherie Calbom, it will seem impossible. So, we'll say to you what Cherie says to them: You've got to get a juicer you'll use, and you've got to use it every day. This is the only way we know that busy people can consume all the fresh fruits and vegetables they need to achieve optimal health.

And there's another reason to juice your produce. Juices make some of the very best dietary supplements available today. They're chock-full of nutrients. We call our drinks "vitamin and mineral cocktails." And if you think you don't need supplements, think again. The American Holistic Medical Association says, "Even if you eat a balanced diet, featuring fresh, whole fruits and vegetables, whole grains and lean proteins, you can still benefit from vitamin and mineral supplements, even if they are not 'necessary' for life. That's because even the best diet from North American farmlands will rarely contain an optimum of nutrients, particularly trace minerals."

But most Americans don't eat a balanced diet. The Standard American Diet (SAD) consists of large amounts of animal products like cheeseburgers, fried chicken, steaks, pizza, and meat-filled sandwiches. We have our favorite snack foods, too, like chocolate chip cookies, pretzels, potato chips and corn chips with dip, cheese and crackers, and bowls of ice cream. We feel lucky to eat anything for breakfast, and at best, it's apt to be a weight-loss breakfast shake consisting mainly of milk and a sweetened protein powder. We try to compensate for our rushed breakfast by eating something healthful at noon from the salad bar, if we're lucky. (But, of course, we cover our salad with heavy, fat-rich dressing.)

All this junk food, excess protein, and fat are hard for the body to digest. For example, the dyes and chemicals used to flavor and preserve that junk food require a lot of extra vitamins and minerals just for the body to metabolize and detoxify them. Junk food is very deficient in nutrients, when it has any at all. So where does the body get the nutrients that are needed for detoxification? From tissues in your body, and most of those tissues have precious few stores. Those chemicals that can't be detoxified get stored in your liver, bones, fat, and other tissues.

Also, the more junk you eat, the more deficient you can become in some nutrients. For example, have you ever wondered why so many people crave sweets? The mineral chromium is involved in the metabolism of sugars. The more sugars you eat, the more chromium you need, but probably you are getting much less than you need because chromium is found mainly in plant foods. Then symptoms of a chromium deficiency develop. One symptom is a craving for sweets, and so the more sweets you eat, the more you crave, until one day you have a full-blown, uncontrollable sugar addiction—and possibly an alarming chromium deficit.

The digestion of proteins and fats also requires a lot of work. Let's look at fat digestion. In the stomach, enzymes mix with fat to break it down into smaller products as it is churned with water and acid. Bile flows from the liver to emulsify the fat mixture in the small intestine. Enzymes flow from the pancreas to further emulsify the fat. Finally, smaller molecules of fatty acids are ready for absorption. The process of protein digestion is equally involved. These processes can take many hours to complete. But it is estimated that fresh fruit and vegetable juices, which are already separated from the fiber, can be assimilated in twenty to thirty minutes because they are so easy to digest and absorb.

Therapeutic Benefits of Fresh Juices

For centuries, fruit and vegetable juices have been used for their therapeutic benefits. The Kentons note that the tradition of raw juice healing goes back to the nineteenth century. At that time, juice-making involved the squeezing of crushed or chopped vegetables through muslin, a very tedious process. Why would anyone go to that much work if the juice did no more for the individual than whole vegetables? It seems that people knew then what some of us are discovering now for the first time: Human beings get well on live juices when nothing else seems to work. This is what Max Gerson, M.D., found when he put his cancer patients on a juice therapy regimen. His "gentle" treatment of cancer is described in detail in his book, *A Cancer Therapy: Results of Fifty Cases.* The fifty people he discusses all recovered from cancer through his natural treatments.

When Norman Walker, D.C., was a young man, he recovered from an illness by eating a raw food and juice diet. He lived to be well over 100, enjoying vibrant health, by practicing what he taught, which was that after the fiber is removed from fruits and vegetables, the remaining juice can be very quickly and easily assimilated. Scores of people got well through his program. Dr. Bircher-Benner discovered the same phenomenon as he worked with many of his patients. It led him to believe there was nothing more therapeutic on Earth than green juice.

To understand juice therapy requires an understanding of juice itself. How would you define juice? We define it as water, flavors, pigments, enzymes, vitamins, minerals, and anutrients. Juice is all these substances working synergistically to give your body the materials that promote healing, energy, and protection from disease. But beyond what we can define, there is a mystery left undefined. It's like the miracle of birth. There is a miracle of energy supplied by live plants that comes from nothing else on this planet. After all is investigated and analyzed, it still can't be fully explained.

We're not saying that juices are "magic bullets." They're not. They should be part of a diet that is a high-quality, junk-free whole-foods plan like the one we recommend in the Basic Diet (see page 285). And juices should be a part of a comprehensive approach to wellness. But what we do know is that juice therapy has worked to bring about recovery from illness for thousands of people, many of whom had been given no hope to live. And for Cherie they did what nothing else could do: they helped her get well. (See her story on page 1.)

Whatever ailments or conditions you are struggling with, we encourage you to make the dietary changes necessary to promote wellness. Get a juicer, if you don't have one already, and use it every day. Make juicing a way of life. Refer to the rest of the book for specifics on your condition. And most of all, don't give up. Healing takes time. Unless you make the necessary changes, you'll never know how good you can feel.

The Western industrialized nations have a large piece of the nutrition puzzle missing from their standard diet. Isn't it time to place the fruit and vegetable pieces in the center of the table, where they belong? Let everything else be the garnishes. It will make a pretty picture from all sides. But, more important, it could help you find the energy you long for, the health you never knew was possible, and the physical appearance you thought belonged only to a fortunate few.

What You Should Know About Juicing

J uicing is the best way we've found to add to your diet the raw fruits and vegetables needed for good health. To most of you, though, juicing is a fairly new idea, and you probably have many questions both about juicing and about nutrition in general. Here are answers to those questions we are most commonly asked.

Juicing separates out the fiber. Don't I need fiber in my diet?

Fiber is essential to health. We encourage you to continue eating all the raw foods you've been eating; in fact, eat more. Fiber is very important to prevent constipation and colorectal cancer. Fiber is not found in animal products, fudge, or potato chips! It is found in fruits, vegetables, whole grains, and legumes. Besides eating these whole foods, drink juices as a supplement for additional nutrients, for protective effects to help your body prevent disease, and for therapeutic benefits. And remember, very few people can find the time to eat enough raw fruits and vegetables to maintain optimal health and energy. Juicing is an easy, quick means to increase your intake of these foods, and it is recommended in addition to a high-fiber diet.

Why can't I just buy bottled, canned, or frozen juice?

Fruits and vegetables take a lot of abuse before they enter a bottle or can. Often, chemicals are poured on them for a variety of reasons. Chemicals can destroy nutrients, and when chemicals are washed off with lots of water, minerals are leached out. Some chemical residues will be left behind for your body to process. Moreover, many juices are heated to high temperatures as a part of pasteurization, which prolongs shelf life. This process kills enzymes, the "spark plugs" of life. Often, additives like sodium benzoate, benzoic acid, sodium nitrate, BHA, and BHT are added. Then the juices go to warehouses, where they may sit for weeks or months before reaching your store. By the time these processed juices get to you, most of the nutrients have been lost. But when you make fresh juice, you're assured of getting a large proportion of nutrients present in the raw fruits and vegetables.

Can't I get all the nutrients I need from vitamin and mineral pills? Why do I need to supplement with fresh juice?

Nutrients in fresh fruits and vegetables are far more potent than those found in pills, because they are paired with "helper nutrients." Nutrients influence each other by working synergistically, meaning they create reactions together within the body. When combined naturally in food, they work much more effectively than when singled out in pill form. But there's another reason as well. Nutrients are continually being discovered and named. For example, you've probably heard of beta-carotene. But how about alpha-carotene? This nutrient has recently shown protective effects against vulvar cancer. And it's found primarily in fruits and vegetables. Or, how about phenols, indoles, aromatic isothiocyanates, terpenes, and organo-sulfur compounds? These strange-sounding substances are part of the new category "anutrients," which, like alpha-carotene, have recently shown protective effects against cancer. And, again, you can find these nutrients in fruits, vegetables, grains, and other plants. If these nutrients are just now being categorized and analyzed, they aren't going to show up in your supplement pills for a while, if ever. But juices provide not only well-known nutrients with identified functions, but also nutrients with roles that are not yet understood or recognized. Finally, if you do need to take a particular supplement, be sure to swallow it with the juices that are highest in that nutrient.

Some people say that fruits and vegetables should not be combined; others say they can be. Is it safe to combine them?

There is no scientific basis for the theory of food combining, which states that fruits and vegetables, starches and proteins, and fruits and proteins should not be combined. But this theory has developed in recent years for a reason. Some people, such as those with impaired digestion, multiple food allergies, or severe fatigue, benefit physically from observing these guidelines. If you experience no adverse symptoms (such as gas, stomachaches, or bloating) from combining these foods, let your taste buds be your guide, and make the combinations you like best.

Are pesticide-sprayed foods harmful?

Exposure to pesticides, herbicides, and other toxic chemicals can contribute to a variety of psychological and neurological symptoms like mental confusion, mental illness, depression, headaches, tingling in the extremities, and abnormal nerve reflexes. These substances are also thought to have given rise to the increased incidence of prostate enlargement seen in the last few decades. Increased cancer rates are also seen in people chronically exposed to such chemicals. We recommend organically grown, unsprayed produce any time you can find it. If it is unavailable in your area, start requesting it from your grocer. When enough requests are made, unsprayed produce will be sold. In the meantime, wash your produce in a biodegradable soap using a vegetable brush to scrub the surfaces well. Rinse thoroughly. This will take care of much of the surface spray. But that which is systemic will appear in the water of the produce and is unavoidable when sprays are used.

How much juice should I drink? Can I get too much?

We recommend several glasses of juice per day. Two to four glasses, in addition to meals, provide good supplementation.

More should be added during a juice fast. Drink a variety of different fruit and vegetable juices to maximize your nutrient intake. We also suggest that you drink at least as much vegetable juice as fruit juice to avoid getting too much fruit sugar. We know of no studies showing adverse effects from too much juice, but common sense is always advisable.

When can I safely start giving juice to my baby?

In the first six months of life, the very best juice for baby is mother's milk. Breastfeeding will provide your baby with many nutritive and protective elements that are not found anywhere else in nature. During this period of time, the baby's digestive system cannot yet handle other foods, including juices. Food allergies can develop when foods are introduced too early in life. But somewhere between six and nine months, when your baby starts showing interest in foods, you can start introducing juices one at a time, observing the suggestions of your pediatrician. Remember to always dilute your baby's juices with equal parts of spring water.

Which parts of fruits and vegetables should not be juiced?

The skins of oranges and grapefruits contain a toxic substance that we don't recommend you drink in large quantities. These skins are also somewhat bitter, so they wouldn't taste good anyway. Apple seeds contain some cyanide, so for that reason we recommend you remove the seeds. Don't juice carrot or rhubarb greens either, again because of the toxicity. Finally, the leaves of celery are often bitter, so you may want to remove them. (For more recipe guidelines, see "Juicing Tips" on page 25.)

JUICING TIPS

It's easy to make fresh juices. All you need are high-quality produce and a good juicer. To get the best results, though, you'll want to keep certain things in mind. The following guidelines will help you prepare juices that are both healthful and delicious.

☐ Whenever you can, use organically grown, unsprayed produce to make the purest juices possible. When organically grown produce isn't available, you may wish to peel the produce before juicing.

☐ Before juicing, wash all produce well, and remove moldy and bruised or otherwise damaged portions of the fruits and vegetables.

☐ Because the skins of oranges and grapefruits contain a toxic substance that should not be consumed in large quantities, and because these skins are somewhat bitter, it's best to peel these fruits before juicing. Leave on the white pithy part of the peel, though; it contains valuable bioflavonoids and vitamin C. Tropical fruits like kiwi and papaya should also be peeled. Often, these fruits have been grown in foreign countries where the use of carcinogenic sprays is still legal. The skins of all other fruits and vegetables, including lemons and limes, may be left on. However, if the produce has been waxed, we recommend removing the peel.

☐ All pits—peach pits, plum pits, etc.—must be removed before juicing. Seeds—lemon and lime seeds, melon seeds, grape seeds, etc.—may be placed in the juicer along with the fruit. However, because apple seeds contain small amounts of cyanide, apple seeds should not be juiced.

☐ When using most produce, don't hesitate to include stems and leaves along with the fruits and vegetables. However, carrot and rhubarb greens should be removed, as they contain toxic substances.

☐ Most fruits and vegetables will have to be sliced or cut into chunks or sticks to accommodate the size of your juicer. After you've used your juicer for a while, you'll know exactly how small the pieces should be.

☐ Most fruits and vegetables have high water contents. This is what makes it possible to juice them. Those fruits and vegetables that contain little water—bananas and avocados, for instance—cannot be placed in the juicer. When using them in your recipes, juice all other fruits first, transfer the juices to a blender, and use the blender to mix in the drier produce.

☐ Most of the recipes in this book will yield a six- to eight-ounce glass of juice. If you desire more servings, double or triple the recipe as necessary. Remember, though, that it's always best to make the juice right before you drink it, rather than making large batches and storing the juice for future use.

PART TWO

The Disorders

Introduction

Part Two contains juice and dietary recommendations for more than fifty common ailments, from acne to wound healing. Each entry offers simple suggestions that will help to make the food you eat work for you and not against you, nourishing your cells and gently supporting them as you move toward health and healing. Much of what is said in these sections will come as no surprise to experienced "juicers." Juicers have known for years what is just now being acknowledged and explained in the scientific literature. But even the old pros will find a few surprises on these pages. Nutrition knowledge is exploding, and each day brings more discoveries that emphasize the importance of fruits and vegetables in the diet.

The juice suggestions and recipes at the end of each entry are designed to fit into one of the diet plans in Part Three. In each Part Two listing, the "Dietary Modifications" section will tell you which diet to follow and what dietary changes to make. Read this segment carefully. It is the foundation upon which the juice suggestions are made. If no diet is mentioned, use the Basic Diet (page 285). Pencil in the recommended juices from Part Two in the blanks provided in the diet plan found in Part Three. This will give you your own personalized juicing program.

If you're new to juicing, be sure to read "Juicing Tips" on page 25 before trying any of the recipes presented in Parts Two and Three. These guidelines will answer many of your questions about preparing produce for use in your juicer, and will help ensure that your juices are both delicious and of the highest quality possible.

Remember that the recommendations in this book should be used only to supplement your physician's recommendations; they should never be used as a replacement for medical care or advice. Also, all of our juice suggestions and recipes will work best when they are incorporated with a total dietary program.

Now, nourish your body to health and healing, and begin to juice for life!

ACNE

Acne is a general term often used to indicate acne vulgaris, which is a chronic inflammatory disease of the sebaceous glands and hair follicles of the skin. It is characterized by blackheads, whiteheads, and pimples. Chronic acne can result in scarring. A contributing factor may be diet, as evidenced by studies of Eskimos and other cultures that first experienced acne after adopting the Western diet. Some acne is caused by a condition known as "skin hypoglycemia" or "skin diabetes." This means that the skin (which is an organ) is intolerant to sugars.

General Recommendations

Cleanse your face at least twice a day with a sulfur-containing soap. After washing, apply benzol peroxide 5-percent gel at night. Extract blackheads every two or three days. Avoid using greasy creams and cosmetics, and avoid medications that contain bromides or iodides.

Dietary Modifications

1. Eliminate sugars. A study has shown that skin glucose tolerance is significantly impaired in acne patients.

2. Eat a high-fiber diet. Acne patients' skin has cleared rapidly when fiber was increased in the diet. Foods high in fiber are fruits, vegetables, whole grain cereals, whole grain breads and crackers, bran, and legumes (beans, lentils, and split peas).

3. Reduce your consumption of fats and junk food. In a study of Eskimos after World War II, it was noted that as the children began consuming the saturated fats and "junk food" of Western society, acne started appearing. The Western diet is too high in calories, fat, salt, and sugar, and too low in vegetables, fruit, and whole grain fiber.

4. *Avoid foods high in trans-fatty acids*. These foods include milk, milk products, margarine, shortening, and hydrogenated vegetable oils. Because milk products are also high in calcium, be sure you are consuming other calcium-rich foods or juices. (See the Calcium-Rich Cocktail at the end of this section.)

5. *Avoid fried foods*.

6. *Eliminate soda pop and artificial sweeteners*.

7. *Limit iodine-containing foods*. Excess iodine consumption can cause an acne-like skin condition. Fast foods have been shown to contain excess quantities of iodine, and many Americans eat far more iodine than they need.

8. *Schedule a cleansing diet for several days to help detoxify your system*. (This is not recommended for anyone under seventeen years of age.) When impurities are not eliminated through the kidneys and bowels fast enough, they can erupt through the skin. A cleansing diet can be very beneficial. (See the Cleansing Diets on page 299.)

9. *Consider the possibility that you have food allergies*. Food allergies can cause skin eruptions in some people. Common allergens include chocolate, milk, refined carbohydrates (sweets), and soft drinks. Note that blood tests are more effective than skin-scratch tests when food allergies are concerned. You might also try the Elimination Diet (see page 296), an effective means of identifying those foods that are causing problems.

10. *Drink no more than one glass of whole milk per day*. The hormones contained in milk can aggravate acne.

11. *A folklore remedy calls for four to five cups of cucumber juice per day for a week*. This is said to purify the blood and lymphatic system, resulting in a clearer complexion.

Nutrients That Help

☐ **Vitamin A** reduces sebum production. Be aware, though, that side effects may result from high doses of supplemental vitamin A. Beta-carotene, found in fresh fruits and vegetables, is a wiser choice. It is converted to vitamin A as needed by your body.

☐ **Vitamin B₆** is beneficial for premenstrual acne breakouts.

☐ **Folic Acid** may be beneficial.

☐ **Selenium with vitamin E** may normalize glutathione peroxidase levels.

☐ **Chromium** improves glucose tolerance levels and enhances insulin sensitivity.

☐ **Zinc** is important in wound healing, inflammation control, and tissue regeneration.

☐ **Essential fatty acids may be helpful, along with a low-fat diet.** Acne sufferers may be deficient in these nutrients. Pure cold-pressed flaxseed oil is a good source of omega-3 fatty acids, as are cold-water fatty fish and green vegetables.

Beneficial Juices

☐ Carrot, kale, and parsley—sources of beta-carotene.

☐ Kale, spinach, and green pepper—sources of vitamin B₆.

☐ Spinach, kale, and beet greens—sources of folic acid.

☐ Red Swiss chard, turnip, and orange—sources of selenium.

☐ Spinach, asparagus, and carrot—sources of vitamin E.

☐ Potato, green pepper, and apple—sources of chromium.

☐ Ginger root, parsley, and carrot—sources of zinc.

☐ Green juices—sources of omega-3 fatty acids (essential fatty acids).

Suggested Juicing Recipes / Acne

Ginger Hopper

¼-inch slice ginger root
4–5 carrots, greens removed
½ apple, seeded

Push ginger through hopper with carrots and apple.

Fresh Complexion Express

2 slices pineapple, with skin
½ cucumber
½ apple, seeded

*Push pineapple through
hopper with cucumber and
apple.*

Energy Shake

Handful parsley
4–6 carrots, greens removed
Parsley sprig for garnish

*Bunch up parsley and push
through hopper with carrots.
Garnish with sprig of parsley.*

Calcium-Rich Cocktail

3 kale leaves
Small handful parsley
4–5 carrots, greens removed
½ apple, seeded

*Bunch up kale and parsley,
and push through hopper
with carrots and apple.*

Green Surprise

1 large kale leaf
2–3 green apples, seeded
Lime twist for garnish

*Bunch up kale leaf and push
through hopper with apples.
Garnish with lime twist. The
surprise is that you won't
taste the kale!*

AGE SPOTS

Age spots, also known as liver spots, are the yellowish-brown
flat spots that appear on the skin as it ages. They are often
caused by free radical change in the skin, and they can be
signals that the body has an accumulation of waste products.

Age spots are caused by poor diet, excess exposure to the sun, impaired liver function, and lack of exercise.

General Recommendations

A comprehensive approach is the most helpful way of getting rid of age spots. Exercise is recommended—regular aerobic exercise at least four times per week for a minimum of thirty minutes each time. Walking is an excellent choice. Limit your exposure to the sun. A folk remedy calls for rubbing castor oil or vitamin E oil on the spots daily. The dietary recommendations that follow are very important as well.

Dietary Modifications

1. Schedule a detoxification plan. See the Cleansing Diets on page 299.

2. Make 50–75 percent of your diet raw foods.

3. Avoid rancid oils. Refrigerate all oils; never store them on a shelf at room temperature once opened. Store all nuts and seeds in the refrigerator or freezer, as they can easily become rancid. Grains should be stored in a cool, dry place. Avoid all fried foods. Hot grease and cooking oils contain high amounts of skin-damaging substances.

4. Avoid sweets, caffeine, alcohol, tobacco, and junk food.

5. Cleanse your liver. Drink beet juice. Two or three ounces of beet juice per day will be sufficient in the beginning of your cleansing program. As you detoxify your liver, you can increase your intake of beet juice to six ounces. Make a tea from one-half teaspoon dandelion root. Start with one cup daily, and increase to two cups per day. If you prefer, try the Seven-Day Liver-Cleansing Diet (see page 312).

Nutrients That Help

☐ **Beta-carotene** is an antioxidant that slows the aging process.

☐ **Vitamin C** is an antioxidant that helps tissue repair.

☐ **Bioflavonoids** work synergistically with vitamin C to repair tissues.

☐ **Vitamin E** is an antioxidant that slows aging and aids in tissue repair.

Beneficial Juices

☐ Carrot, kale, parsley, and spinach—sources of beta-carotene.

☐ Kale, parsley, green pepper, and spinach—sources of vitamin C.

☐ Grape, cherry, grapefruit, and lemon—sources of bioflavonoids. (For a more extensive list, see AGING in Part Two.)

☐ Spinach, asparagus, and carrot—sources of Vitamin E.

Suggested Juicing Recipes / Age Spots

Beauty Spa Express

Small handful parsley Handful spinach 4–5 carrots, greens removed ½ apple, seeded	*Bunch up parsley and spinach, and push through hopper with carrots and apple.*

Fresh Complexion Express

2 slices pineapple, with skin ½ cucumber ½ apple, seeded	*Push pineapple through hopper with cucumber and apple.*

Cherie's Cleansing Cocktail

¼-inch slice ginger root 1 beet ½ apple, seeded 4 carrots, greens removed	*Push ginger, beet, and apple through hopper with carrots.*

Garden Salad Special

3 broccoli flowerets
1 garlic clove
4–5 carrots or 2 tomatoes
2 stalks celery
½ green pepper

Push broccoli and garlic
through hopper with carrots
or tomatoes. Follow with
celery and green pepper.

Morning Tonic

1 grapefruit, peeled (leave
    white pithy part)
1 apple, seeded

Push grapefruit through
hopper with apple.

AGING

Aging is not a disease, although many people think it is. The good news is that premature aging doesn't have to happen. While no magic elixir exists to reverse this process, research has shown that certain nutrients can help to slow the onset of visible signs of aging, can prevent many disorders, and can extend life expectancy.

General Recommendations

Our Standard American Diet (SAD) accounts for the five leading causes of disease in America. It also contributes to accelerated aging more than any other single factor. The SAD is high in refined carbohydrates, cholesterol, saturated fats, and processed foods. It is low in vegetables, fruits, whole grains, legumes, seeds, and nuts—all of which provide dietary fiber and most of our anti-aging vitamins and minerals.

In addition to the SAD's overload of foods that tax the body and insufficient quantities of foods that feed the body, this diet also harms us by increasing the number of substances that are known as free radicals. Free radicals are produced within

our bodies, are obtained from the environment, and are ingested with our food. In our food supply, they come from
pesticides; fried, barbecued, and charbroiled foods; alcohol;
coffee; and additives. Free radicals are highly reactive
molecules that can damage cells. This cell-damaging process
leads to many disorders and contributes to aging, as well. Free
radicals need to be detoxified, and the anti-aging nutrients like
Vitamins C and E, beta-carotene, and the mineral selenium
are found primarily in fruits and vegetables—foods that are in
scarce supply in the Standard American Diet.

Clearly, a different diet is needed. Leslie and Susannah
Kenton, in their book *Raw Energy*, state that raw foods have
an enormous potential for improving not only a person's
appearance but also the quality of his or her life. For example,
they cite the fact that uncooked foods are one reason why many
health spas attract so many people. Two weeks on a raw diet,
they note, make a person look years younger, with firmer flesh;
softer facial lines; and skin, eyes, and hair that glow with
vibrant health. Two years on a diet high in raw foods can
completely transform a person's shape, and often can restore
health, as well. If that's not enough to get you excited about
raw foods, we guess you probably just don't get excited!

Dietary Modifications

*1. Eat a diet that's rich in raw fruits and vegetables and
their juices.* Ideally, 50 percent of the diet should be composed
of raw foods.

*2. Increase the amount of gel-forming fiber in your diet
by boosting your intake of flaxseeds; oat and rice bran;
and pectins, which are found in fruits and vegetables.*

3. Try adding black currant juice to your diet. This juice,
which is rich in bioflavonoids, has been shown to promote
longevity.

*4. Eat more cabbage, yogurt, and olive oil, all of which
have been shown to increase longevity.*

*5. Try adding thyme and lavender to dishes. These herbs
have been used traditionally to slow down the aging
process.*

6. Reduce your consumption of refined foods such as white flour and its products. Yes, there goes your favorite sourdough bread, the morning donut, and the white-flour pasta! But the rewards are plentiful for eating whole grain breads, rolls, and pastas.

7. Avoid refined sugar and its products. This includes chocolate chip cookies, frozen yogurt, and your favorite candy bars. But think about the lines you won't get on your face because you said, "No"!

8. Reduce your intake of saturated fats, cholesterol, and animal proteins. And here's a surprise: butter is better than margarine. There are substances in margarine that have been shown in studies to contribute to cancer. You can finally say that there is something that tastes better *and* is actually better for you. But don't celebrate with too much butter. The general guideline is no more than about four tablespoons of saturated fat per day.

9. Make one or two days a week vegetarian. Try making your main courses on these days from beans, lentils, split peas, and soybean products like tofu. In addition, use more of these vegetable proteins in your daily diet.

10. Select only cold-processed or expeller-pressed vegetable oils, and increase your intake of fish oils.

11. Choose nutritious snacks such as nuts, seeds, nut or seed butters, raw vegetable sticks, whole grain crackers, popcorn without butter, and fresh fruit.

12. Reduce caffeine by eliminating or limiting your consumption of coffee, black tea, and chocolate.

13. Significantly reduce or avoid alcohol.

14. Avoid all processed foods as much as possible.

15. Incorporate a detoxification program into your lifestyle. Use the Juice Fast or another effective cleansing diet to eliminate the toxins from your body. (See the Cleansing Diets on page 299.)

Nutrients That Help

☐ **Vitamins C and E and the mineral selenium** are antioxidants that protect the cells from free-radical damage, thus preventing premature aging. In other words, antioxidants gobble up the bad guys before they get your cells.

☐ **Beta-carotene and other carotenoids (over 500 have been identified)** are antioxidants that are converted by the body to vitamin A as needed. These are some of the most powerful interceptors known to protect the body from a particular free-radical bad guy called singlet oxygen. The carotenoids are also very helpful in preventing shrinkage of the thymus gland, and thus strengthening the immune system.

☐ **Bioflavonoids** prevent free-radical damage. Like the carotenoids, these nutrients, which are found in plants, are considered antioxidants.

☐ **Methionine and cysteine** are sulfur-containing amino acids that may promote longevity. Sulfur is abundant in beans, fish, liver, eggs, brewer's yeast, cabbage, and nuts.

Beneficial Juices

☐ Kale, parsley, green pepper, and broccoli—sources of vitamin C.

☐ Spinach, asparagus, and carrot—sources of vitamin E.

☐ Red Swiss chard, turnip, garlic, and orange—sources of selenium.

☐ Carrot, kale, parsley, and spinach—sources of beta-carotene and other carotenoids.

☐ Apricot, black currant, blackberry, broccoli, cabbage, cantaloupe, cherry, grape, grapefruit, lemon, orange, papaya, parsley, plum, prune, sweet pepper, and tomato—sources of bioflavonoids.

Suggested Juicing Recipes / Aging

Beauty Spa Express

Small handful parsley
Handful spinach
4–5 carrots, greens removed
½ apple, seeded

*Bunch up parsley and
spinach, and push through
hopper with carrots and
apple.*

Fresh Complexion Express

2 slices pineapple, with skin
½ cucumber
½ apple, seeded

*Push pineapple through
hopper with cucumber and
apple.*

High-Calcium Drink

3 kale leaves
Small handful parsley
4–5 carrots, greens removed

*Bunch up kale and parsley,
and push through hopper
with carrots.*

Garden Salad Special

3 broccoli flowerets
1 garlic clove
4–5 carrots or 2 tomatoes
2 stalks celery
½ green pepper

*Push broccoli and garlic
through hopper with carrots
or tomatoes. Follow with
celery and green pepper.*

Cantaloupe Shake

½ cantaloupe, with skin

*Cut cantaloupe in strips, and
push through hopper.*

Fruit Salad Cocktail

1 medium bunch grapes
½ apple, seeded
¼ lemon

*Push grapes through hopper,
followed by apples and lemon.*

ALLERGIES

An allergy is a reaction to a substance that in nonsensitive persons would produce no effect. It is an antibody-antigen reaction that may be caused by the release of histamine or histamine-like substances from injured cells. The offending substance is known as an allergen and can be anything that brings on the symptoms of an allergy.

General Recommendations

Food allergies should be identified, and problem foods should be avoided. Blood tests are more effective than the skin-scratch test in identifying food allergies. Or try the Elimination Diet (page 296), which is a self-test for allergies, and is the oldest and most reliable test known for identifying food allergens. Certain additives, such as aspartame (NutraSweet), monosodium glutamate (MSG), and sulfites, can also cause allergic reactions. In addition, an overgrowth of the yeast known as *Candida albicans* can cause a variety of food sensitivities. Either a blood test or stool culture can determine whether there is a yeast overgrowth present in the body. When this yeast overgrowth is brought under control, many people notice that their allergies and sensitivities have improved. (*See* CANDIDIASIS in Part Two for the appropriate diet.) In addition, the Juice Fast (page 301) has been helpful for many allergy sufferers.

Dietary Modifications

1. Identify food allergies and eliminate those foods that cause symptoms. You may wish to follow the Elimination Diet. (See page 296.)

2. Avoid additives that commonly cause reactions, including MSG, sulfites, and aspartame (NutraSweet).

3. Follow the Immune Support Diet. (See page 293.)

4. Refer to Sally Rockwell's Allergy Recipes *for cooking ideas.* She has also prepared a self-help survival kit for allergy sufferers, titled *The Rotation Game.*

Nutrients That Help

☐ **Vitamin B6** may be beneficial for MSG sensitivity.

☐ **Vitamin B12** may have therapeutic benefits. Speak to your doctor about supplementation, as this nutrient cannot be obtained from juices.

☐ **Vitamin C** may reduce blood histamine levels and MSG sensitivity.

☐ **Vitamin E** has antihistamine activity.

☐ **Molybdenum** may be helpful, as this nutrient might be deficient in the majority of people with sulfite sensitivity.

☐ **Lactobacillus acidophilus and Lactobacillus bifidus** may be beneficial, as a deficiency may exist with food allergies. Speak to your doctor about supplementation, as these substances are not found in juices.

☐ **Bioflavonoids** potentiate the action of vitamin C.

Beneficial Juices

☐ Kale, spinach, and sweet pepper—sources of vitamin B6.
☐ Kale, parsley, and collard greens—sources of vitamin C.
☐ Spinach, asparagus, and carrot—sources of vitamin E.
☐ Cauliflower, spinach, and garlic—sources of molybdenum.
☐ Orange, cantaloupe, and parsley—sources of bioflavonoids.

Suggested Juicing Recipes / Allergies

Vitamin E-Rich Drink

Small handful spinach
4–5 carrots, greens removed
3–4 asparagus spears

Bunch up spinach and push through hopper with carrots and asparagus.

Molybdenum Drink

Small handful spinach
1 garlic clove
4–5 carrots, greens removed
4 small cauliflower buds

Bunch up spinach with garlic, and push through hopper with carrots and cauliflower.

Cherie's Cleansing Cocktail

¼-inch slice ginger root
1 beet
½ apple, seeded
4 carrots, greens removed

Push ginger, beet, and apple through hopper with carrots.

Cantaloupe Shake

½ cantaloupe, with skin

Cut cantaloupe in strips, and push through hopper.

ALOPECIA

See HAIR LOSS.

ALZHEIMER'S DISEASE

Alzheimer's disease, also called presenile dementia, is similar to senile dementia but occurs in the forty-to-sixty-year age group.

This condition is characterized by memory loss, severe mood swings, personality changes, inability to concentrate, inability to communicate, and distorted perception of time and space. Autopsies of Alzheimer's victims have revealed large amounts of aluminum and silicon in the neurofibrillary tangles and senile plaques of the brain. Excesses of calcium, bromine, and sulfur have also been found. In addition, Alzheimer's victims have been found to be deficient in potassium, selenium, boron, zinc, and vitamin B_{12}. At this time, the only "cure" is prevention.

General Recommendations

Because of the association of Alzheimer's disease with excessive amounts of aluminum in the brain, it is recommended that all sources of aluminum be removed from daily use. Such substances include aluminum-contaminated drinking water, buffered aspirin, certain antacids, various douches, many underarm antiperspirants, some makeup, certain brands of toothpaste, diarrhea medications, dandruff shampoos, aluminum containers such as beer cans, aluminum foil, and aluminum-containing baking powder.

To prevent this disease or halt early-stage progression, regular blood tests that measure mineral and heavy-metal levels are recommended. Hair analysis is effective in identifying heavy metals like aluminum. Based on your test results, you and your doctor can take measures to correct deficiencies and eliminate excesses.

Dietary Modifications

1. Follow the Basic Diet. (See page 285.)

2. Avoid fast foods, especially those prepared with processed cheese. Most processed cheese contains aluminum. Fried foods should be avoided as well because of toxic substances known as free radicals produced in the frying process.

3. Avoid foods and drinks that were cooked or stored in aluminum containers or pots.

4. Eat a high-fiber diet.

5. Schedule a Juice Fast (see page 301) several times a year, or use the Six-Week Cleansing Diet (page 313) once a year to help cleanse the body of heavy metals.

6. Include mackerel, sardines, and salmon in your diet, as these foods are rich in coenzyme Q_{10}, an antioxidant that enhances oxygen transport to cells.

7. Eat sulfur-rich foods such as onions, garlic, beans, and eggs. These foods help cleanse the body of heavy metals. Soluble fibers such as pectin, guar gum, psyllium seed, and oat bran are also helpful detoxifying agents.

8. See also MEMORY LOSS in Part Two.

Nutrients That Help

☐ **Beta-carotene** is an antioxidant that helps the body detoxify.

☐ **Vitamin C** is an antioxidant that destroys free radicals.

☐ **Bioflavonoids** enhance vitamin C's effectiveness and help circulation.

☐ **Vitamin E** is an antioxidant that improves circulation and tissue repair.

☐ **Selenium** is an antioxidant that helps the body detoxify.

Beneficial Juices

☐ Carrot, kale, parsley, and spinach—sources of beta-carotene.

☐ Kale, parsley, green pepper, and spinach—sources of vitamin C.

☐ Grape, cherry, grapefruit, and lemon—sources of bio-flavonoids. (See AGING in Part Two for a more extensive list.)

☐ Spinach, asparagus, and carrot—sources of vitamin E.

☐ Turnip, garlic, and orange—sources of selenium.

Suggested Juicing Recipes /
Alzheimer's Prevention

Potassium Broth

Handful parsley
Handful spinach
4–5 carrots, greens removed
2 stalks celery

*Bunch up parsley and
spinach leaves, and push
through hopper with carrots
and celery.*

Very Veggie Cocktail

Handful wheatgrass
½ handful parsley
Handful watercress
4 carrots, greens removed
3 stalks celery
½ cup chopped fennel
½ apple, seeded

*Bunch up wheatgrass,
parsley, and watercress, and
push through hopper with
carrots, celery, fennel, and
apple.*

Cherie's Cleansing Cocktail

¼-inch slice ginger root
1 beet
½ apple, seeded
4 carrots, greens removed

*Push ginger, beet, and apple
through hopper with carrots.*

Spring Tonic

Handful parsley
4 carrots, greens removed
1 garlic clove
2 stalks celery

*Bunch up parsley and push
through hopper with carrots,
garlic, and celery.*

Fruit Salad Cocktail

1 medium bunch grapes
½ apple, seeded
¼ lemon

*Push grapes through hopper,
followed by apples and lemon.*

ANEMIA

Anemia is a condition in which there is a reduction in the total number of red blood cells or volume of blood, or an abnormal size or shape of red blood cells. It is characterized by extreme paleness, weakness, a tendency to tire easily, insomnia, irritability or depression, and decreased resistance to infection. Iron is an important factor in anemia, as the formation of red blood cells is impaired in those lacking sufficient amounts of iron. However, there are many causes of anemia; iron deficiency is only one. Other deficiencies, including those of folic acid and vitamin B_{12}, along with abnormal hemoglobin production as in sickle cell anemia, may also cause this condition.

General Recommendations

Effective treatment of anemia depends on the type of anemia. The three most common types are iron deficiency, folic acid deficiency, and vitamin B_{12} deficiency anemia. Treatment involves supplying the body with the appropriate nutrients in an absorbable form. If you suspect you are anemic, we suggest you seek medical advice.

Dietary Modifications

1. For all anemias, eat a diet high in green leafy vegetables and their juices. Other iron-rich foods that should be consumed in quantity include beans, blackstrap molasses, dried apricots, raisins, almonds, and shellfish. Vitamin C has been shown to significantly enhance the absorption of iron. Calf liver is no longer recommended unless it was organically grown (without hormones or antibiotics) in a fairly pollution-free environment. The liver is the organ where toxins are stored. Eating liver today could do more harm than good. Black tea should also be avoided, because it contains tannins that can reduce iron absorption as much as 50 percent when taken with meals.

2. It is recommended that vitamin B₁₂ always be taken along with folic acid. Foods rich in folic acid include black-eyed peas, wheat germ, lean meat, beans, bran, asparagus, lentils, walnuts, spinach, and kale. Foods rich in vitamin B₁₂ include clams, oysters, sardines, egg yolks, trout, salmon, tuna, and lean meat.

3. If a vitamin B₁₂ deficiency anemia exists because of a lack of an intrinsic factor (a substance produced in the stomach), fairly large doses of vitamin B₁₂ are needed, and medical supervision is recommended.

Nutrients That Help

Iron Deficiency Anemia

☐ Iron.

☐ Vitamin C.

Folic Acid Deficiency Anemia

☐ Folic Acid.

☐ Vitamin B₁₂.

Vitamin B₁₂ Deficiency Anemia

☐ Folic Acid.

☐ Vitamin B₁₂.

Beneficial Juices

☐ Parsley, beet greens, and carrot—sources of iron.

☐ Kale, parsley, and green pepper—sources of vitamin C.

☐ Asparagus, spinach, and kale—sources of folic acid.

☐ There are no fruits or vegetables rich in vitamin B₁₂. For strict vegetarians, vitamin B₁₂ supplementation may be necessary. Or try eating vitamin B₁₂-fortified cereal two or three times a week.

Suggested Juicing Recipes / Anemia

Folic Acid Special

2 kale leaves   *Bunch up kale, parsley, and*
Small handful parsley   *spinach, and push through*
Small handful spinach   *hopper with carrots.*
4–5 carrots, greens removed

Iron-Rich Drink

3 beet tops   *Bunch up beet tops, and push*
4–5 carrots, greens removed   *through hopper with carrots,*
½ green pepper   *followed by green pepper and*
½ apple, seeded   *apple.*

Spring Tonic

Handful parsley   *Bunch up parsley and push*
4 carrots, greens removed   *through hopper with carrots,*
1 garlic clove   *garlic, and celery.*
2 stalks celery

Popeye's Favorite

Small handful spinach   *Bunch up spinach and push*
4–5 carrots, greens removed   *through hopper with carrots*
½ apple, seeded   *and apple.*

ANXIETY

See STRESS.

APPETITE, POOR

See UNDERWEIGHT.

ARTHRITIS

Arthritis is inflammation of a joint usually accompanied by pain and, frequently, changes in structure. The most common forms of arthritis are osteoarthritis and rheumatoid arthritis.

OSTEOARTHRITIS

Osteoarthritis is a form of arthritis affecting the bones and joints. It is characterized by mild early-morning stiffness, stiffness after periods of rest, pain that is worse when the joint is used, and loss of joint function. Symptoms can range from local tenderness, swelling of soft tissues, bony swelling, and restricted mobility, to cracking of joints in movement. Osteoarthritis is divided into two categories—primary and secondary. Primary osteoarthritis is a degenerative condition brought about by wear and tear on the body. Secondary osteoarthritis is brought about by predisposing factors such as trauma or previous inflammatory disease of the joint.

General Recommendations

Osteoarthritis sufferers should achieve and maintain normal body weight. Excess weight places an added strain on the weight-bearing joints. For some individuals, symptoms disappear completely after weight loss. (See the Weight-Loss Diets on page 319.)

Dietary Modifications

1. Try eliminating the nightshade family—tomatoes, peppers, potatoes, eggplant, and tobacco. If symptoms improve even slightly, continue to avoid these foods. Though not proven, there is a theory that a long-term low-level consumption of the solanum alkaloids found in this family inhibits normal collagen repair in the joints or encourages inflammatory degeneration of the joints.

2. Avoid the citrus family—lemons, limes, oranges, and grapefruits. This family, like the nightshade family, is thought to contribute to joint swelling.

3. Avoid all refined foods such as white flour, white sugar, and preserved and processed foods. Eat a nutritious diet that emphasizes whole grains, legumes (beans, split peas, and lentils), seeds, nuts, vegetables, and fruits, and includes only a small portion of low-fat animal products.

4. Significantly decrease your consumption of sweets and alcohol.

5. Consider testing for food allergies.

6. Check for hydrochloric acid deficiency. Seek medical advice in this regard.

7. Try a juice fast, which has been shown to be very helpful for arthritis. See page 301 for more information.

Nutrients That Help

☐ **Niacinamide** may bring a noticeable improvement within two to six weeks. This nutrient is said to be especially beneficial for degenerative arthritis of the knee. (*Warning!* Niacinamide supplements may affect the liver or cause nausea.)

☐ **Pantothenic acid** may be helpful, as a deficiency of this nutrient has been associated with osteoarthritis.

☐ **Vitamin C** may be beneficial.

☐ **Vitamin E** may produce effects similar to those of non-steroidal anti-inflammatory drugs.

☐ **Methionine** is important in cartilage structures.

☐ **Superoxide dismutase** may have therapeutic benefits.

☐ **Copper** may be helpful, as a deficiency of this nutrient has been associated with osteoarthritis.

☐ **Bioflavonoids** have been shown to be beneficial.

☐ **Bromelain** has anti-inflammatory properties.

Beneficial Juices

☐ Broccoli and kale—sources of pantothenic acid.

☐ Kale, parsley, and spinach—sources of vitamin C.

☐ Spinach and carrot—sources of vitamin E.

☐ Carrot, ginger root, and apple—sources of copper.

☐ Cherry and blueberry—sources of bioflavonoids.

☐ Pineapple—the only source of bromelain.

Suggested Juicing Recipes / Osteoarthritis

Garden Salad Special

3 broccoli flowerets
1 garlic clove
4–5 carrots or 2 tomatoes
2 stalks celery
½ green pepper

Push broccoli and garlic through hopper with carrots or tomatoes. Follow with celery and green pepper.

Digestive Special

Handful spinach
4–5 carrots, greens removed

Bunch up spinach and push through hopper with carrots.

Bromelain Special

¼ pineapple, with skin

Push pineapple through hopper.

Ginger Hopper

¼-inch slice ginger root   *Push ginger through hopper*
4–5 carrots, greens removed   *with carrots and apple.*
½ apple, seeded

Gingerberry Fizz

1 quart blueberries   *Push blueberries through*
1 medium bunch grapes   *hopper, followed by grapes*
¼-inch slice ginger root   *and ginger. Pour juice into*
Sparkling water   *ice-filled glass. Fill glass to*
                                  top with sparkling water.

RHEUMATOID ARTHRITIS

Rheumatoid arthritis is a systemic disease characterized by inflammatory changes in joints and related structures. Its symptoms include fatigue, low-grade fever, weakness, and joint stiffness and pain. There is often severe joint pain, with increased inflammation beginning in small joints and progressively affecting all joints in the body. Evidence exists that rheumatoid arthritis is an autoimmune reaction in which antibodies develop against components of joint tissues.

Dietary Modifications

1. Consume a low-fat, low-calorie diet excluding most animal sources (meat, dairy products, and so forth). Studies have shown that patients following this type of diet experienced remission of joint symptoms. A vegetarian diet, excluding all animal sources but fish, has been found to be very beneficial.

2. Increase your consumption of cold-water fish, e.g., mackerel, salmon, tuna, and sardines. Cod-liver oil may also be beneficial.

3. Exclude refined sugar, refined wheat flour, corn flour, salt, strong spices, alcohol, tea, and coffee from your diet.

4. Identify food allergies. (See the Elimination Diet on page 296.)

5. Check for low stomach acid (hydrochloric acid). See your doctor for testing.

6. One folk remedy calls for drinking basil as a tea. Basil has been used to ease rheumatoid pain.

7. Try a juice fast, which has been shown to help arthritis. See page 301 for more information.

Nutrients That Help

☐ **Vitamin C** has anti-inflammatory action.

☐ **Vitamin E** has anti-inflammatory action.

☐ **Vitamin K** may stabilize the membranes and cells of rheumatoid tissue.

☐ **Pantothenic acid** may be helpful, as deficiencies of this nutrient have been found to be directly related to symptoms.

☐ **Copper** has anti-inflammatory action.

☐ **Iron** may be helpful, as an iron deficiency may be involved. (Supplementation is controversial. Food is the best source.)

☐ **Manganese** may have therapeutic benefits.

☐ **Selenium** may be helpful, as a deficiency may be involved.

☐ **Sulfur** may be helpful, as a deficiency may be involved.

☐ **Zinc** may be helpful, as a deficiency may be involved.

☐ **Bromelain** has anti-inflammatory properties.

☐ **Omega-3 fatty acids** have therapeutic benefits.

☐ **Superoxide dismutase** has anti-inflammatory properties.

Beneficial Juices

☐ Parsley, broccoli, and spinach—sources of vitamin C.

☐ Spinach, carrot, and tomato—sources of vitamin E.

☐ Broccoli, lettuce, and cabbage—sources of vitamin K.

☐ Broccoli and kale—sources of pantothenic acid.

☐ Carrot, ginger root, and apple—sources of copper.

☐ Parsley, beet greens, and broccoli—sources of iron.

☐ Spinach, beet greens, carrot, turnip, orange, and grape—sources of manganese.

☐ Ginger root, parsley, and carrot—sources of selenium.

☐ Cabbage and kale—sources of sulfur.

☐ Ginger root, parsley, garlic, and carrot—sources of zinc.

☐ Pineapple—the only source of bromelain.

☐ Dark green vegetables—sources of omega-3 fatty acids.

Suggested Juicing Recipes / Rheumatoid Arthritis

Popeye's Favorite

Small handful spinach
4–5 carrots, greens removed
½ apple, seeded

Bunch up spinach and push through hopper with carrots and apple.

Potassium Broth

Handful parsley
Handful spinach
4–5 carrots, greens removed
2 stalks celery

Bunch up parsley and spinach leaves, and push through hopper with carrots and celery.

Bromelain Special

¼ pineapple, with skin

*Push pineapple through
hopper.*

Garden Salad Special

3 broccoli flowerets
1 garlic clove
4–5 carrots or 2 tomatoes
2 stalks celery
½ green pepper

*Push broccoli and garlic
through hopper with carrots
or tomatoes. Follow with
celery and green pepper.*

Ginger Hopper

¼-inch slice ginger root
4–5 carrots, greens removed
½ apple, seeded

*Push ginger through hopper
with carrots and apple.*

Maureen's Spicy Tonic

¼ pineapple, with skin
½ apple, seeded
¼-inch slice ginger root

*Push pineapple through
hopper with apple and ginger.*

Gingerberry Fizz

1 quart blueberries
1 medium bunch grapes
¼-inch slice ginger root
Sparkling water

*Push blueberries through
hopper, followed by grapes
and ginger. Pour juice into
ice-filled glass. Fill glass to
top with sparkling water.*

Cherie's Cleansing Cocktail

¼-inch slice ginger root
1 beet
½ apple, seeded
4 carrots, greens removed

*Push ginger, beet, and apple
through hopper with carrots.*

ASTHMA

Asthma is defined as difficulty in breathing accompanied by sporadic wheezing sounds caused by a spasm of the bronchial tube or a swelling of the mucous membranes. It is characterized by shortness of breath, coughing, and expelling of mucus. Two types of asthma have been identified. One condition is caused by allergens, while the other develops without any specific allergens being found. In all cases, but particularly in the latter, emotions must be considered, as stress may cause or worsen asthmatic attacks.

Dietary Modifications

1. According to recent studies, a vegetarian diet has been found to be helpful for the majority of asthmatics. The recommended diet excludes all meat, fish, eggs, and dairy products. (For children, especially, professional nutritional counseling is recommended to ensure that the vegetarian diet includes adequate protein during critical growth years. This is important for teen-agers also.)

2. Limit all animal products. The production of substances that contribute to the allergic and inflammatory reactions found in asthma come from arachidonic acid, a fatty acid found mainly in animal products.

3. Drink pure spring water rather than chlorinated tap water.

4. Eliminate all coffee, tea, chocolate, sugar, and salt.

5. Every day, be sure to eat large portions of raw fruits and vegetables.

6. Limit or eliminate all cereals except for buckwheat and millet.

7. Identify all food allergies. Particularly in infants and children, elimination diets (the identification of allergens by eliminating foods on a trial basis) have been successful in the treatment of asthma. Some of the most common allergens include milk, chocolate, wheat, citrus fruits, food colorings, eggs, fish, shellfish, and nuts, particularly peanuts. (See the Elimination Diet on page 296 for further details.)

8. Remove all food additives from the diet. Many preservatives and dyes have been reported to cause asthma attacks. Examples of additives include tartrazine, benzoates, sulfur dioxide, and, particularly, sulfites.

9. Generously include onions and garlic in your diet, unless allergic, as they have been found to ward off an enzyme that generates an inflammatory chemical.

10. Chili pepper has been used naturopathically to break an asthma attack. This food has been shown to have components that desensitize the airways to various irritants.

11. In one study, the diet had to be followed for one year before some of the participants experienced full benefits. "Don't give up too soon!" is the moral of this story.

12. For adults (not children under seventeen) a juice fast is recommended. (See page 301 for further details.)

13. Low stomach acid may be a contributing factor. See your doctor for testing.

14. Avoid using aspirin and other nonsteroidal anti-inflammatory drugs, as they can bring on an asthma attack.

15. Try one of these four folk remedies:

- Mix two tablespoons of lemon juice with water, and drink before meals.

- Make ginger tea by juicing a piece of ginger and simmering it in water. If desired, add a little honey or lemon juice for taste. Drink before meals.

- Juice one red onion and mix with a small amount of honey. Take one teaspoon every hour during an attack.

- During an asthma attack, put your hands in hot—*not scalding*—water.

Nutrients That Help

☐ **Vitamin B6** may be deficient in asthmatics. This supplement has been shown to decrease frequency and severity of wheezing and asthma attacks.

☐ **Vitamin B12** may be deficient in asthmatics. With the addition of vitamin B12, patients in one study showed less shortness of breath during exertion. Speak to your doctor about supplementation, as this nutrient cannot be obtained from juices.

☐ **Vitamin C** is an antioxidant that can provide an important defense against bronchial constriction.

☐ **Beta-carotene** is effective in healing the epithelial lining of the respiratory tract.

☐ **Vitamin E** is an antioxidant that can inhibit the formation of inflammatory compounds.

☐ **Selenium** is effective in inhibiting the production of leukotrienes, substances that stimulate bronchial constriction.

☐ **Magnesium** relaxes the bronchial muscle.

Beneficial Juices

☐ Kale, spinach, and turnip greens—sources of vitamin B6.

☐ Kale, parsley, broccoli, and spinach—sources of vitamin C.

☐ Carrot, collard greens, kale, and parsley—sources of beta-carotene and other carotenoids.

☐ Spinach, asparagus, and carrot—sources of vitamin E.

☐ Red Swiss chard, turnip, garlic, and orange juice—sources of selenium.

☐ Beet greens, spinach, parsley, and garlic—sources of magnesium.

Suggested Juicing Recipes / Asthma

Digestive Special

Handful spinach
4–5 carrots, greens removed

Bunch up spinach and push through hopper with carrots.

Energy Shake

Handful parsley
4–6 carrots, greens removed
Parsley sprig for garnish

Bunch up parsley and push through hopper with carrots. Garnish with sprig of parsley.

Magnesium Drink

1 garlic clove
Small handful parsley
4–5 carrots, greens removed
2 stalks celery
Parsley sprig for garnish

Wrap garlic in parsley, and push through hopper with carrots and celery. Pour juice into glass, and garnish with sprig of parsley.

Vegetable Cocktail

1 garlic clove or small piece
    of onion
3 broccoli flowerets
2 kale leaves
5 carrots, greens removed
Dash cayenne pepper
Seasoning(s) of choice

Roll garlic (or onion) and broccoli in kale leaves, and push through hopper with carrots. Add pepper. Season to taste.

ATHEROSCLEROSIS

Atherosclerosis is a disorder characterized by a hardening and thickening of the blood vessels caused by accumulations of fat-containing materials called plaque within or beneath the surface of the blood vessels. This condition is often associated with high blood pressure and a weak pulse. Symptoms can include angina, leg cramps, gradual mental deterioration, weakness, or dizziness.

General Recommendations

While diet may be the most important contributor to atherosclerosis, other lifestyle factors also play an important part in the prevention or reversal of this condition. Physical exercise has a direct relationship to cholesterol levels. Engage in some aerobic exercise, such as walking, at least three times a week. If you don't have a dog to walk, rent one! Smoking greatly increases your risk and should be stopped. Stress management is also a must, even if you're a "type B" personality.

Dietary Modifications

1. Follow the Basic Diet (see page 285), which is low in fat and high in fiber.

2. Reduce dietary cholesterol.

3. Reduce fats, especially animal fats and hydrogenated vegetable oils (e.g., margarine, which is often promoted as beneficial). Try making Better Butter by combining a pound of butter with one cup expeller-pressed vegetable oil, like safflower or sunflower oil.

4. Increase your consumption of vegetable proteins such as soybeans, lentils, and split peas. Soybeans are especially beneficial, as they are rich in lecithin, a nutrient that enhances the solubility of cholesterol and actually aids in pulling cholesterol from tissue deposits.

5. Avoid coffee and alcohol. Epidemiological studies have correlated coffee consumption with atherosclerosis and hyperlipidemia. Alcohol has been shown to have a harmful effect on blood pressure, body weight, and glucose tolerance.

6. Increase your consumption of omega-3 fatty acids by eating more cold-water fish and fish oils and adding flax-

seed oil to your diet. Pure cold-pressed flaxseed oil is the highest in omega-3 fatty acids and is excellent for the prevention and care of atherosclerosis. Try to have one-half tablespoon each day.

7. Eat more garlic, ginger, and onions, all of which have been shown to reduce the likelihood of blood-clot formation.

8. Add alfalfa sprouts—and their juice—to your diet. Alfalfa has been shown to decrease cholesterol levels and help shrink the fatty plaque that can block blood vessels.

Nutrients That Help

☐ **Vitamin B₆** deficiency is associated with a higher risk of atherosclerosis. This nutrient may inhibit blood clots from forming, and can play an important role in preventing this condition.

☐ **Vitamin C** may be deficient in sufferers of atherosclerosis. Supplementation may lower total cholesterol, triglycerides, and total fats while elevating the level of high-density lipoproteins (HDLs), which sweep the body clean of excess cholesterol.

☐ **Vitamin E** may help prevent platelets from clumping together and forming blood clots, may lower cholesterol, and may decrease pain in limbs caused by inadequate blood supply.

☐ **Niacin**, although long used to lower cholesterol, is no longer recommended as a supplement except under strict medical supervision. In supplemental form it is often toxic, causing liver damage and glucose intolerance. There is no worry of high-dose toxicity, however, when you ingest foods that are rich in niacin. Niacin is highest in brewer's yeast, rice bran, wheat bran, turkey, chicken, and trout.

☐ **Bromelain** is recommended to inhibit blood-clot formation, relieve angina, and break down fatty plaques.

☐ **Calcium** lowers cholesterol and triglycerides and prevents blood clots.

☐ **Copper** deficiency can elevate cholesterol. Typical American diets are low in copper.

☐ **Chromium** has been shown to lower cholesterol and triglycerides. Most Americans consume an inadequate amount of chromium, causing a number of problems, including a craving for sweets. (*See* CRAVINGS in Part Two for more information.)

☐ **Magnesium** deficiency has been associated with an increased risk of heart disease. Supplementation may reduce total cholesterol, raise HDL cholesterol, and prevent the formation of blood clots.

☐ **Potassium** may inhibit the formation of fatty plaque deposits.

☐ **Selenium** deficiency is correlated with atherosclerosis. Supplementation may prevent blood clots from forming.

☐ **Lecithin** enhances the solubility of cholesterol. Soybeans are high in lecithin.

Beneficial Juices

☐ Kale, spinach, turnip greens, and sweet pepper—sources of vitamin B6.

☐ Kale, parsley, green pepper, and broccoli—sources of vitamin C.

☐ Spinach, asparagus, and carrot—sources of vitamin E.

☐ Pineapple—the only source of the enzyme bromelain.

☐ Kale, collard greens, turnip greens, and parsley—sources of calcium.

☐ Carrot, garlic, and ginger root—sources of copper.

☐ Potato, green pepper, apple, and spinach—sources of chromium.

☐ Beet greens, spinach, parsley, and garlic—sources of magnesium.

☐ Parsley, Swiss chard, spinach, and garlic—sources of potassium.

☐ Red Swiss chard, turnip, garlic, and orange—sources of selenium.

Suggested Juicing Recipes / Atherosclerosis

Ginger Hopper

¼-inch slice ginger root
4–5 carrots, greens removed
½ apple, seeded

Push ginger through hopper with carrots and apple.

High-Calcium Drink

---

3 kale leaves
Small handful parsley
4–5 carrots, greens removed

Bunch up kale and parsley, and push through hopper with carrots.

Garden Salad Special

---

3 broccoli flowerets
1 garlic clove
4–5 carrots or 2 tomatoes
2 stalks celery
½ green pepper

Push broccoli and garlic through hopper with carrots or tomatoes. Follow with celery and green pepper.

Potassium Broth

Handful parsley
Handful spinach
4–5 carrots, greens removed
2 stalks celery

Bunch up parsley and spinach leaves, and push through hopper with carrots and celery.

BACKACHE

Backache is a common syndrome characterized by pain and tenderness in the muscles or in the muscles' attachments to other regions, such as the sacroiliac. Back pain is a signal that something is wrong in the body. It can be caused by infection, disorders of the vertebral column, or a number of other conditions, including stress. Back pain is a sign to take action and seek professional medical advice. There are some things you can do in addition to help the healing process.

General Recommendations

From a psychological standpoint, much can be done to help control back pain. For example, focusing, relaxation methods, and biofeedback can all be very helpful. In addition, physical therapy, massage, and acupuncture have provided therapeutic benefits. Diet may not have much influence on how one perceives back pain, but it can be very important in the healing process. An exception would be certain herbal remedies that have been used throughout history in the treatment of pain, such as red pepper, clove oil, German chamomile, and wintergreen oil. Traditionally, chestnuts also have been used to relieve backache.

Dietary Modifications

1. Follow the Basic Diet. (See page 285.)

2. Reduce your consumption of animal fats. In decreasing your consumption of these fats, you will decrease your intake of arachidonic acid, which contributes to the inflammatory process.

3. Eat more fatty cold-water fish, such as mackerel, herring, and salmon. These fish contain a substance that has anti-inflammatory properties.

4. Avoid instant coffee. A study has shown that instant coffee blocks certain receptor sites in the brain that naturally help the body control pain. When these receptor sites are blocked, the body is more susceptible to pain.

5. Follow one of the cleansing diets. (See page 299.) Many people have experienced pain relief and healing from injuries during and after a cleansing diet. Cherie experienced a great deal of pain after a car accident in which she sustained whiplash injuries. After six months of therapy without much improvement, she went on a three-day juice fast, after which her condition greatly improved.

Nutrients That Help

☐ **Vitamin K** has shown some promising results in pain management in studies not yet published.

☐ **Copper** deficiency can contribute to pain perception.

☐ **D-phenylalanine,** an amino acid, may effectively ease chronic pain even when medications offer no relief. Speak to your doctor about supplementation.

Beneficial Juices

☐ Turnip greens, broccoli, lettuce, cabbage, and spinach—sources of vitamin K.

☐ Carrot, garlic, and ginger root—sources of copper.

Suggested Juicing Recipes / Backache

Vegetable Express

2 lettuce leaves
1 small wedge cabbage
4–5 carrots, greens removed
3 broccoli flowerets
½ apple, seeded

Bunch up lettuce leaves, and push through hopper with cabbage, carrots, broccoli, and apple.

Ginger Hopper

¼-inch slice ginger root
4–5 carrots, greens removed
½ apple, seeded

*Push ginger through hopper
with carrots and apple.*

Digestive Special

Handful spinach
4–5 carrots, greens removed

*Bunch up spinach and push
through hopper with carrots.*

Ginger Fizz

¼-inch slice ginger root
1 apple, seeded
Sparkling water

*Push ginger through hopper
with apple. Pour juice into
ice-filled glass. Fill glass to
top with sparkling water.*

Potassium Broth

Handful parsley
Handful spinach
4–5 carrots, greens removed
2 stalks celery

*Bunch up parsley and
spinach leaves, and push
through hopper with carrots
and celery.*

BALDNESS

See HAIR LOSS.

BLADDER INFECTION (CYSTITIS)

Bladder infection is medically termed cystitis. It is a condition
in which the bladder is invaded by a microorganism that

multiplies and produces inflammation. The symptoms of this infection include burning pain when urinating, frequent urges to urinate, excessive urination at night, dark or strong-smelling urine, and lower abdominal pain.

Dietary Modifications

1. Follow the Immune Support Diet. (See page 293.)

2. Drink large amounts of fluids. At least sixteen ounces of unsweetened cranberry juice should be consumed per day. You can make it yourself with fresh cranberries, adding fresh apples to sweeten it naturally. If cranberries are not available in your store, purchase cranberry juice concentrate from a health food store and add it to fresh apple juice. Since it is a concentrate, one tablespoon is adequate for thirty-two ounces of apple juice. (If this mixture is too strong, lessen the amount of cranberry concentrate the next time and add more apple juice now.) There is a substance in cranberry juice that coats the bacteria so that it can't stick to your bladder and cause infection. In addition, cranberry juice acidifies urine, inhibiting bacterial growth.

3. A folk remedy calls for drinking one-half cup of pomegranate juice mixed with one-half cup of water twice a day.

4. Avoid all sweets in any form, including health food store cookies. Dilute all fruit juices with water, except for your homemade cranberry-apple juice. Avoid all refined carbohydrates, including white bread, regular pizza dough, and regular pasta.

5. Include generous amounts of garlic and onions in your diet. These foods have antimicrobial activity that can help fight infection.

6. Try goldenseal extract, an effective herbal antimicrobial agent.

Nutrients That Help

☐ **Vitamin C** has protective effects against infection and strengthens the immune system.

☐ **Beta-carotene** helps strengthen immunity and protects against infection.

☐ **Bioflavonoids** enhance the absorption of Vitamin C and have an antibacterial effect.

☐ **Zinc** promotes a healthy immune system.

Beneficial Juices

☐ Kale, parsley, green pepper, and broccoli—sources of vitamin C.

☐ Carrot, collard greens, parsley, and spinach—sources of beta-carotene.

☐ Cantaloupe, black currant, papaya, and lemon—sources of bioflavonoids.

☐ Ginger root, parsley, garlic, and carrot—sources of zinc.

☐ Cranberry—contains "the cranberry factor," which inhibits bacterial growth.

☐ Pomegranate—this juice is a folk remedy for cystitis.

Suggested Juicing Recipes / Bladder Infection

Cranberry Cocktail

½ cup cranberries
3–4 apples, seeded (add more apples if too sour)

Push cranberries through hopper with apples. If fresh or frozen cranberries are not available, use 1 Tbsp. cranberry juice concentrate to 32 oz. apple juice.

Ginger Fizz

¼-inch slice ginger root
1 apple, seeded
Sparkling water

Push ginger through hopper
with apple. Pour juice into
ice-filled glass. Fill glass to
top with sparkling water.

Ginger Hopper

¼-inch slice ginger root
4–5 carrots, greens removed
½ apple, seeded

Push ginger through hopper
with carrots and apple.

Garden Salad Special

3 broccoli flowerets
1 garlic clove
4–5 carrots or 2 tomatoes
2 stalks celery
½ green pepper

Push broccoli and garlic
through hopper with carrots
or tomatoes. Follow with
celery and green pepper.

Cantaloupe Shake

½ cantaloupe, with skin

Cut cantaloupe in strips, and
push through hopper.

BLOOD CLOTS

See THROMBOSIS.

BRONCHITIS

Bronchitis is the inflammation of the mucous membranes of
the air passages (bronchi). It is characterized by chills, malaise,

soreness and constriction behind the sternum (breastbone), incessant coughing, breathing difficulty, and slight fever.

General Recommendations

Bed rest and steam inhalations are recommended. Large amounts of liquids should be consumed, including diluted vegetable juices, soups, and herbal teas. A heating pad or hot-water bottle placed on the chest and back for thirty minutes per day may be helpful. For information on botanical medicines, a mustard poultice, natural cough syrups, and posture drainage, see the *Encyclopedia of Natural Medicine* by Michael Murray and Joseph Pizzorno.

Dietary Modifications

1. Follow the Immune Support Diet. (See page 293.)

2. Reduce sugar consumption, including fruit sugars, to no more than 50 grams of simple carbohydrates. Sugars depress the immune system. One piece of fruit contains 15 grams; therefore, no more than about three pieces of fruit per day should be eaten, with no added sweeteners.

3. Limit dairy consumption. Milk tends to thicken mucus.

4. Increase your intake of fluids.

5. A traditional remedy calls for adding the juice of two lemons and two teaspoons of honey to a pint of flaxseed tea. Take one teaspoon of this mixture every half hour during the acute phase.

Nutrients That Help

☐ **Vitamin C** strengthens the immune system, helping the body to fight infections.

☐ **Bioflavonoids** enhance the absorption of vitamin C.

☐ **Beta-carotene** strengthens the immune system.

☐ **Zinc lozenges** promote a healthy immune system.

☐ **Bromelain** has anti-inflammatory properties.

Beneficial Juices

☐ Kale, parsley, green pepper, and broccoli—sources of vitamin C.

☐ Tomato, parsley, sweet pepper, and lemon—sources of bioflavonoids. (See AGING in Part Two for a more extensive list.)

☐ Carrot, kale, parsley, and spinach—sources of beta-carotene.

☐ Ginger root, parsley, garlic, and carrot—sources of zinc.

☐ Pineapple—the only source of bromelain.

Suggested Juicing Recipes / Bronchitis

Ginger Hopper

¼-inch slice ginger root
4–5 carrots, greens removed
½ apple, seeded

Push ginger through hopper with carrots and apple.

Bromelain Special

¼ pineapple, with skin

Push pineapple through hopper.

Garden Salad Special

3 broccoli flowerets
1 garlic clove
4–5 carrots or 2 tomatoes
2 stalks celery
½ green pepper

Push broccoli and garlic through hopper with carrots or tomatoes. Follow with celery and green pepper.

Energy Shake

Handful parsley
4–6 carrots, greens removed
Parsley sprig for garnish

*Bunch up parsley and push
through hopper with carrots.
Garnish with sprig of parsley.*

Ginger Tea

2-inch slice ginger root
¼ lemon
1 pint water
1 stick cinnamon, broken
4–5 cloves
Dash nutmeg or cardamom

*Juice ginger and lemon. Place
juice in saucepan, and add
water, cinnamon, and cloves.
Gently simmer. Add nutmeg
or cardamom.*

Ginger Fizz

¼-inch slice ginger root
1 apple, seeded
Sparkling water

*Push ginger through hopper
with apple. Pour juice into
ice-filled glass. Fill glass to
top with sparkling water.*

BRUISING

A bruise is an injury that does not break the skin but does cause the rupture of small underlying blood vessels, resulting in a discoloration of the skin. Easy bruising that occurs with no apparent injuries is due to fragile capillaries.

Dietary Modifications

1. Generously include foods high in vitamin C, bioflavonoids, and vitamin E.

2. Follow the Basic Diet. (See page 285.)

Nutrients That Help

☐ **Vitamin C** protects against bruising by strengthening capillary walls.

☐ **Bioflavonoids** work synergistically with vitamin C to prevent easy bruising.

☐ **Vitamin E** works synergistically with vitamin C to repair tissues.

Beneficial Juices

☐ Kale, parsley, green pepper, and broccoli—sources of vitamin C.

☐ Apricot, black currant, blackberry, broccoli, cabbage, cantaloupe, cherry, grape, grapefruit, lemon, orange, papaya, parsley, plum, prune, sweet pepper, and tomato—sources of bioflavonoids.

☐ Spinach, asparagus, and carrot—sources of vitamin E.

Suggested Juicing Recipes / Bruising

Garden Salad Special

---

3 broccoli flowerets
1 garlic clove
4–5 carrots or 2 tomatoes
2 stalks celery
½ green pepper

Push broccoli and garlic through hopper with carrots or tomatoes. Follow with celery and green pepper.

Potassium Broth

Handful parsley
Handful spinach
4–5 carrots, greens removed
2 stalks celery

Bunch up parsley and spinach leaves, and push through hopper with carrots and celery.

Orange Delight

2–3 oranges, peeled (leave
    white pithy part)
½ apple, seeded

*Push oranges and apples
through hopper.*

Fruit Cocktail

1 large bunch grapes
2 apples, seeded
1 lemon wedge

*Push grapes, apples, and
lemon through hopper.*

BURSITIS

Bursitis is the inflammation of a bursa, a small, fluid-filled, pad-like sac or cavity found in connecting tissues, usually in the vicinity of a joint. Bursitis is especially common in those bursae located between bony prominences and muscles or tendons, as in the shoulder or knee. This condition is characterized by symptoms of severe pain in the affected joint, especially during movement. There is also a limited range of motion. Bursitis may be a secondary condition as a result of trauma, strain, infection, or arthritis. If the bursa develops calcified deposits, it can become a chronic problem.

General Recommendations

After any injury or sprain, immediate treatment is very important. The **RICE** approach should be followed:

Rest the area that was injured.

Ice should be applied to the painful area to reduce swelling and bleeding.

Compress the injured area with an elastic bandage to limit swelling and bleeding.

Elevate the body part above heart level to increase drainage of fluids from the damaged area.

Physical therapy may be very helpful, including trans-cutaneous electrical nerve stimulation and ultrasound. After the acute phase, begin doing range-of-motion exercises with proper guidance. Seek medical advice regarding appropriate treatments.

Dietary Modifications

1. Follow the Basic Diet. (See page 285.)

2. A folk remedy calls for eating one avocado each day until the pain subsides.

Nutrients That Help

☐ **Vitamin B12**, administered in intramuscular injections, provided relief of pain and caused considerable reabsorption of calcium deposits in one study. See your doctor regarding injections or supplementations, as this nutrient cannot be obtained from juice.

☐ **Vitamin C** is important in the prevention and repair of injuries.

☐ **Beta-carotene** is needed for wound healing and the synthesis of collagen, a protein that forms connective tissue.

☐ **Vitamin E** speeds wound healing.

☐ **Bioflavonoids** are helpful in stabilizing collagen structures and in reducing inflammation. Quercetin is particularly effective.

☐ **Zinc** speeds wound healing.

☐ **Bromelain**, the enzyme in pineapple, is an effective anti-inflammatory agent.

Beneficial Juices

☐ Kale, parsley, green pepper, and broccoli—sources of vitamin C.

☐ Carrot, collard greens, kale, and parsley—sources of beta-carotene.

☐ Spinach, asparagus, and carrot—sources of vitamin E.

☐ Grape, cantaloupe, lemon, and orange (citrus fruits without outer peel but with white pithy part)—rich sources of bioflavonoids. (For a more extensive list of the bioflavonoids, see AGING in Part Two.)

☐ Ginger root, parsley, garlic, and carrot—sources of zinc.

☐ Pineapple—the only source of the enzyme bromelain.

Suggested Juicing Recipes / Bursitis

Fruit Cocktail

1 large bunch grapes   *Push grapes through hopper*
2 apples, seeded   *with apples and lemon.*
1 lemon wedge

Watercress Express

Handful watercress   *Bunch up watercress and*
4–5 carrots   *push through hopper with*
3 radishes   *carrots and radishes.*

Cantaloupe Shake

½ cantaloupe, with skin   *Cut cantaloupe in strips, and*
                              push through hopper.

Ginger Hopper

¼-inch slice ginger root   *Push ginger through hopper*
4–5 carrots, greens removed   *with carrots and apple.*
½ apple, seeded

Garden Salad Special

---

3 broccoli flowerets
1 garlic clove
4–5 carrots or 2 tomatoes
2 stalks celery
½ green pepper

Push broccoli and garlic through hopper with carrots or tomatoes. Follow with celery and green pepper.

Orange Delight

2–3 oranges, peeled (leave white pithy part)
½ apple, seeded

Push oranges and apples through hopper.

CANCER

Cancer refers to any of the various types of malignant growths and to the illnesses caused by them. Cancer occurs when a cell or group of cells escapes homeostatic control—a state of equilibrium produced by a balance of functions within the body—and reproduces at will, showing abnormal growth patterns. Factors such as diet, stress, chemical carcinogens, ionizing radiation, viruses, hormones, heredity, and chronic irritation have all been shown to play a part in causing cancer. Researchers estimate that 80 to 90 percent of all cancers are environmentally related. In that broad category termed "environmental," the National Cancer Institute lists diet as the number-one contributing factor.

General Recommendations

Because of the seriousness and complexity of this disease, it is far beyond the scope of this book to cover even the extent of dietary recommendations for cancer. Some very basic guidelines will be given for dietary modifications and therapeutic nutrients. We refer you to *A Cancer Therapy* by

Max Gerson, M.D., and *The Famous Bristol Detox Diet* by Alec Forbes, M.D., for further information on diet and cancer. *The Cancer Prevention Diet* by Michio Kushi approaches relief of the disease from a macrobiotic focus. Kushi's diet involves a complete philosophy that is different from the raw-foods approach that we and the other authors mentioned have taken. However, it offers many practical suggestions that are worth trying for specific types of cancer, and these suggestions can be incorporated into the raw-foods-and-juices regimen.

We encourage you to make major changes in your diet if you have cancer. There is a common notion that once someone has cancer, there is little that can be done nutritionally to reverse the situation. Research and clinical experience do not support that position, however. We know that when someone is ill, the supply of nutrients must be increased for his or her body to get well. It is very difficult for healing to take place on a diet consisting of gelatin desserts (high in sugar and artificial ingredients), fish sticks (high in saturated fat), milk shakes (high in sugar and fat), or any of the other nutrient-deficient foods that are part of our Standard American Diet. In her practice as a clinical nutritionist, Cherie has seen many cancer patients who wanted to "play" at dietary changes, and their health suffered from that game. We encourage you to make the recommended dietary changes a way of life right now. You have nothing to lose—except, perhaps, some fat-rich junk foods.

Be aware that chemotherapy, radiation, and surgery can weaken the immune system, as does the cancer itself. When the immune system is weakened, one is more susceptible to candidiasis, a yeastlike fungal overgrowth that will further weaken this system. See CANDIDIASIS in Part Two for further details, and seek appropriate medical advice as needed. A healthy immune system will enable the body to fight the cancer. It is only through strong immunity that recovery can actually take place.

To prevent cancer, dietary changes are imperative. Our cultural eating patterns are known to contribute to the five leading causes of disease in America, of which cancer is number two. A staggeringly large number of research studies now show that a good diet, more than any other factor, can prevent this disease. For example, beta-carotene has been shown to prevent cancer through its ability to scavenge free radicals and inhibit the production of new cancer cells. Beta-carotene is found in deep yellow, green, or red fruits and vegetables, and is converted by the body to Vitamin A as needed. But we may not be able to eat adequate amounts of beta-carotene-rich foods in a day. In addition, when we are under stress, our diets become even more inadequate because our nutritional needs increase. Supplementation is the current recommendation. A pint or more of carrot juice daily may be our best protection against cancer.

Dietary Modifications

1. Follow the Immune Support Diet. (See page 293.)

2. Specifically avoid all foods that have been linked with cancer. These foods include hydrogenated vegetable oils (including margarine), sugars of all kinds, caffeine, milk and its products (except for a small amount of plain yogurt), animal proteins (except for a little fish occasionally), food additives, peanuts and peanut butter, and alcoholic beverages, as well as fried, barbecued, and smoked foods.

3. Include generous amounts of freshly made vegetable juices to feed the body with nutrient-dense foods.

4. Eat a daily serving of vegetables from the cruciferous family. This includes Brussels sprouts, cabbage, broccoli, cauliflower, kale, and turnips. Cruciferous vegetables contain substances known as glucosinolates, which help the body neutralize and excrete certain carcinogens.

5. Include fish oils and other oils high in omega-3 fatty acids. Pure expeller- or cold-pressed flaxseed oil is highest in this nutrient. (Buy only oil that has been refrigerated in opaque bottles.) All of these oils have been found in studies to reduce the growth rate of breast tumors.

6. Consume generous amounts of ginger root, garlic, and onions, all shown in studies to have cancer-fighting properties.

7. Incorporate a juice cleansing fast as part of your diet design. The juice therapy regimen was the central part of

Dr. Max Gerson's treatment and is discussed in his book *A Cancer Therapy*. (See the Juice Fast, page 301.)

Nutrients That Help

☐ **Beta-carotene** is an antioxidant that has demonstrated potent abilities to inhibit the rapid production of new cancer cells.

☐ **Vitamin C** is an antioxidant that converts free radicals to harmless waste and is said to detoxify carcinogenic compounds.

☐ **Vitamin E** is an antioxidant and free-radical scavenger. It has been shown in studies to inhibit tumor growth and enhance the effects of cytoxic drugs (drugs that block the growth of cells in the body), allowing a reduction of the dosage.

☐ **Selenium** is one of the antioxidants that protect cell membranes and enhance the immune system, possibly inhibiting cancer growth.

☐ **Calcium, potassium, and chromium** deficiencies are associated with a variety of cancers.

Beneficial Juices

☐ Carrot, collard greens, kale, parsley, and spinach—sources of beta-carotene.

☐ Kale, parsley, green pepper, and broccoli—sources of vitamin C.

☐ Spinach, asparagus, and carrot—sources of vitamin E.

☐ Red Swiss chard, turnip, garlic, and orange—sources of selenium.

☐ Collard greens, turnip greens, kale, parsley, dandelion greens, watercress, and beet greens—sources of calcium.

□ Parsley, Swiss chard, garlic, and spinach—sources of potassium.

□ Potato, green pepper, apple, and spinach—sources of chromium.

Suggested Juicing Recipes / Cancer

Ginger Hopper

¼-inch slice ginger root 4–5 carrots, greens removed ½ apple, seeded	*Push ginger through hopper with carrots and apple.*

Garden Salad Special

3 broccoli flowerets 1 garlic clove 4–5 carrots or 2 tomatoes 2 stalks celery ½ green pepper	*Push broccoli and garlic through hopper with carrots or tomatoes. Follow with celery and green pepper.*

Potassium Broth

Handful parsley Handful spinach 4–5 carrots, greens removed 2 stalks celery	*Bunch up parsley and spinach leaves, and push through hopper with carrots and celery.*

Cherie's Cleansing Cocktail

¼-inch slice ginger root 1 beet ½ apple, seeded 4 carrots, greens removed	*Push ginger, beet, and apple through hopper with carrots.*

Garlic Express

Handful parsley
1 garlic clove
4–5 carrots, greens removed
2 stalks celery

*Bunch up parsley and push
through hopper with garlic,
carrots, and celery.*

Cantaloupe Shake

½ cantaloupe, with skin

*Cut cantaloupe in strips, and
push through hopper.*

Alkaline Special

¼ head cabbage (red or
     green)
3 stalks celery

*Push cabbage and celery
through hopper.*

Chlorophyll Cocktail

3 beet tops
Handful parsley
Handful spinach
4 carrots, greens removed
½ apple, seeded

*Bunch up beet tops, parsley,
and spinach, and push
through hopper with carrots
and apple.*

Calcium-Rich Cocktail

3 kale leaves
Small handful parsley
4–5 carrots, greens removed
½ apple, seeded

*Bunch up kale and parsley,
and push through hopper
with carrots and apple.*

CANDIDIASIS

Candidiasis is an infection of any species of Candida (the most
common of which is *Candida albicans*), which is a yeastlike

fungus. It can affect any system in the body, but primarily it affects the gastrointestinal, nervous, endocrine, and immune systems. It is characterized by symptoms of chronic fatigue, low energy, loss of sex drive, and malaise. Symptoms connected with the gastrointestinal tract include bloating, gas, intestinal cramps, rectal itching, changes in bowel functions, and thrush ("white carpet" on the tongue). Nervous system problems include depression, poor memory, irritability, and inability to concentrate. Genitourinary system complaints include vaginal yeast infections and frequent bladder infections. Endocrine system problems include premenstrual syndrome (PMS) and other menstrual problems. Immune system complaints include lowered immunity, allergies, and chemical sensitivities.

Candida overgrowth is often caused by overuse of antibiotics. Antibiotics kill both harmful and friendly bacteria. It is the friendly bacteria that keep the Candida under control. Candida overgrowth can also be the result of using other drugs, such as oral contraceptives, anti-ulcer drugs, and corticosteroids; of digestive disorders; or of excessive sugar intake. If you suspect that you have Candida, you can take an extensive written quiz in the *Encyclopedia of Natural Medicine* by Michael Murray and Joseph Pizzorno, or a brief quiz in *The Yeast Connection* by William G. Crook. If your score warrants further testing, see your doctor for a stool culture test to measure Candida overgrowth or a blood test to measure Candida antibodies.

General Recommendations

Digestive secretions like hydrochloric acid, pancreatic enzymes, and bile help prevent the overgrowth of Candida. It is important to find out if you have low levels of these secretions and to correct any deficiencies with supplements of HCl betaine, pancreatic enzymes, and substances that encourage bile flow. Naturopathic doctors are excellent resources for this type of treatment.

Your liver may be a key to overcoming *Candida albicans*. Animal studies have shown that poor liver function encourages Candida overgrowth. Candida also manufactures a type of alcohol that can cause its sufferers to feel constantly "hung over." This puts a strain on the liver, which must continually detoxify the alcohol. When your liver is overloaded with toxins, it is not able to filter blood properly. This becomes an even greater problem when you attempt to kill off the Candida, causing additional toxins to be released into your blood stream. Thus, support and cleansing of the liver is a vital part of Candida treatment.

Although an outline of the complete treatment for candidiasis is beyond the scope of this book, dietary and nutrient guidelines are given. After reading the dietary recommendations, you may feel that there is nothing left to eat. Cherie thought that, too, in the beginning. But there's a lot you can do with the foods allowed. We suggest buying a copy of *The Yeast Connection Cookbook* by William G. Crook and Marjorie Hurt Jones; *The Coping With Candida Cookbook* by Sally Rockwell; or *Candida: A Twentieth Century Disease* by Shirley S. Lorenzani for recipes and meal-planning guidelines.

Once you get rid of this yeast overgrowth, we don't recommend going back to your old ways of eating. Chances are strong that the "yeasties" will start taking over again. Cherie tried more than once to eat the old junk-food diet, or even a high-carbohydrate diet, and learned the hard way that the anti-Candida diet outlined below works best for maintenance, too.

Dietary Modifications

1. Avoid refined sugar, including sucrose and fructose. Sugars weaken the immune system. And Candida finds sweets to be a delectable delight! If you want to get well, you can't feed those little yeasties. That means no more sweets and a limitation of all carbohydrates. Also, be aware of those desserts that say "sugar-free." They often contain fructose or some other sweetener. In addition, no other sweets should be eaten, including fruit juice concentrate, honey, molasses, maple syrup, malt barley syrup, and fruit juices. That's right—*no fruit juice.* Also, all dried fruits must be avoided because of sugar and mold content. You'll just have to pull that proverbial sweet tooth. But don't be too discouraged. There is a reward for all this. It's called *health.*

2. Limit your intake of fresh fruit to one serving per day of only the following fruits—apples, blueberries and other berries, cherries, and pears. You may add some of your allowable fruit serving each day to your juice recipes. For example, you can use a few slices of apple to sweeten your vegetable drinks. But remember to subtract that amount from the *one* serving of fruit you would eat that day.

3. Avoid all canned or frozen juices. All vegetable juices should be freshly made. Most canned and frozen juices contain citric acid, a by-product of yeast, which can provoke reactions.

4. Avoid milk and its products, except for butter and a small portion of plain yogurt (about one-half cup per day). Keep in mind that milk sugars, like other sugars, promote yeast growth. (For extra calcium, see the High-Calcium Drink at the end of this section.)

5. Limit your servings of wheat, oats, rye, barley, corn, rice, potatoes, and millet to about one-half to one cup per meal. Servings should total no more than about four to five per day, and only whole grains may be consumed.

6. Limit your intake of yeasts and molds, which are found in commercial breads, rolls, and most crackers. Yeast-free breads can be purchased at many health food stores and co-ops. Beer, wine, and other alcoholic beverages also contain yeast, as do salad dressings, vinegars, pickles, sauerkraut, relishes, green olives, commercial soups, potato chips, and dry-roasted nuts. Many vitamin and mineral supplements also include yeasts. Purchase only those labeled "yeast-free."

7. Avoid pickled, smoked, and dried meats, fish, and poultry. This includes smoked salmon, oysters, sardines, hot dogs, salami, corned beef, ham, bacon, and pastrami.

8. Avoid peanuts and peanut butter because of their high content of aflatoxins, a carcinogenic mold.

9. Foods that can be eaten generously include all vegetables (except for those specified), legumes, fish, poultry, lean meat, seeds, and nuts. Wash all vegetables well in a biodegradable soap, and rinse before eating.

10. For snacks, try seeds, nuts, and nut butters (except for peanuts).

11. Include generous amounts of garlic in your diet. Garlic has shown excellent antifungal properties.

12. Use the spices ginger and cinnamon and the herbs thyme and rosemary in your foods, as these seasonings contain very powerful anti-Candida agents.

13. Avoid herbal teas because of the molds, but include Pau d'arco tea. This tea has shown potent Candida-killing effects.

14. Cleanse your liver with the Seven-Day Liver-Cleansing Diet. (See page 312.) Be sure, though, to omit all fruits.

Nutrients That Help

☐ **Vitamin B6** is necessary in the production of hydrochloric acid and aids in immune function.

☐ **Selenium** protects the immune system.

☐ **Iron** is required for energy production and a healthy immune system.

☐ **Zinc** promotes a healthy immune system and protects the liver.

☐ **Lactobacillus acidophilus** helps restore the friendly intestinal bacteria. Speak to your doctor about supplementation, as this substance is not found in juices.

☐ **Fiber supplements (guar gum, pectin, and psyllium seeds)** promote elimination and healthy bowel function.

Beneficial Juices

☐ Kale, spinach, and turnip greens—sources of vitamin B6.

☐ Red Swiss chard, turnip, garlic, and radish—sources of selenium.

☐ Parsley, beet greens, dandelion greens, and broccoli—sources of iron.

☐ Ginger root, parsley, garlic, and carrot—sources of zinc.

Suggested Juicing Recipes / Candidiasis

Ginger Hopper

¼-inch slice ginger root
4–5 carrots, greens removed
½ apple, seeded

Push ginger through hopper with carrots and apple.

Garden Salad Special

3 broccoli flowerets
1 garlic clove
4–5 carrots or 2 tomatoes
2 stalks celery
½ green pepper

Push broccoli and garlic through hopper with carrots or tomatoes. Follow with celery and green pepper.

Potassium Broth

Handful parsley
Handful spinach
4–5 carrots, greens removed
2 stalks celery

Bunch up parsley and spinach leaves, and push through hopper with carrots and celery.

Immune Builder

Handful parsley
1 garlic clove
5 carrots, greens removed
3 stalks celery

Bunch up parsley, and push through hopper with garlic, carrots, and celery.

Cherie's Cleansing Cocktail

¼-inch slice ginger root
1 beet
½ apple, seeded
4 carrots, greens removed

Push ginger, beet, and apple through hopper with carrots.

Energy Shake

Handful parsley
4–6 carrots, greens removed
Parsley sprig for garnish

*Bunch up parsley and push
through hopper with carrots.
Garnish with sprig of parsley.*

Digestive Special

Handful spinach
4–5 carrots, greens removed

*Bunch up spinach and push
through hopper with carrots.*

High-Calcium Drink

---

3 kale leaves
Small handful parsley
4–5 carrots, greens removed

*Bunch up kale and parsley,
and push through hopper
with carrots.*

CANKER SORES

Canker sores are painful white spots on the mucous membranes of the mouth. They occur most often in females, and they are contagious. This is a common condition, estimated to affect more than 20 percent of the population. The cause appears to be related to stress, candidiasis, food sensitivities, poor dental hygiene, or nutrient deficiencies.

General Recommendations

It is important to identify any food sensitivities. A blood test may be helpful in this process, or you can try the Elimination Diet (see page 296). There is a high incidence of canker sores in patients with celiac disease—an inability to digest the gluten of some grain foods. But even when celiac disease is not present, a person who is prone to canker sores may be more sensitive to gluten (in wheat, oats, rye, and barley) and may need to limit the intake of these foods. Again, the Elimination Diet may be helpful in determining this sensitivity.

If you suspect that you have candidiasis (see CANDIDIASIS in Part Two), you may want to get a blood or stool test to check for that condition. Also, if you notice a higher incidence of canker sores in times of great stress, a relaxation program may be beneficial. Deficiencies in the nutrients iron, vitamin B_{12}, and folic acid can also contribute to canker sores. You may want to see a nutritionally oriented health professional for recommendations on supplementation. And, if you do take supplements, swallow them with juices highest in those nutrients to gain maximum benefits.

Dietary Modifications

1. Eat a diet low in animal products. Animal protein produces excess acid in the body, contributing to the occurrence of canker sores.

2. Avoid sweets and citrus fruits, all refined and processed foods, and coffee.

3. Consume generous amounts of cultured milk products (yogurt, kefir, cottage cheese, or buttermilk), garlic, and onions.

4. Eliminate chewing gum and lozenges.

Nutrients That Help

☐ **Iron** deficiencies can cause canker sores.

☐ **Folic acid** deficiencies can cause canker sores.

☐ **Vitamin B_{12}** deficiencies can cause canker sores. Speak to your doctor about supplementation, as this nutrient cannot be obtained from juices.

☐ **Zinc** is beneficial if serum levels are low.

☐ **Beta-carotene** speeds the healing of mucous membranes.

Beneficial Juices

☐ Parsley, beet greens, broccoli, and spinach—sources of iron.

☐ Kale, spinach, beet greens, and cabbage—sources of folic acid.

☐ Ginger root, parsley, garlic, and carrot—sources of zinc.

☐ Carrot, kale, parsley, and spinach—sources of beta-carotene.

Suggested Juicing Recipes / Canker Sores

Ginger Hopper

¼-inch slice ginger root
4–5 carrots, greens removed
½ apple, seeded

Push ginger through hopper with carrots and apple.

Popeye's Favorite

Small handful spinach
4–5 carrots, greens removed
½ apple, seeded

Bunch up spinach and push through hopper with carrots and apple.

Folic Acid Special

2 kale leaves
Small handful parsley
Small handful spinach
4–5 carrots, greens removed

Bunch up kale, parsley, and spinach, and push through hopper with carrots.

Iron-Rich Drink

3 beet tops
4–5 carrots, greens removed
½ green pepper
½ apple, seeded

Bunch up beet tops, and push through hopper with carrots, followed by green pepper and apple.

CARDIOVASCULAR DISEASE

See ATHEROSCLEROSIS; CHOLESTEROLEMIA; CIRCULATION PROBLEMS; HYPERTENSION; THROMBOSIS.

CARPAL TUNNEL SYNDROME

Carpal tunnel syndrome is defined as pressure on the median nerve at the point where it goes through the carpal tunnel of the wrist. It is characterized by soreness, tenderness, and weakness of the muscles of the thumb, as well as numbness, tingling, and burning in the first three fingers of the hand. These symptoms are experienced most often at night. This condition is usually found in people who perform repetitive movements with their hands, such as office workers or carpenters. Other causes include injuries to the wrist, inflammation, rheumatoid arthritis, swelling, some systemic diseases, and nutrient deficiency.

General Recommendations

It is important to remove the cause of this condition if at all possible. For some, this may involve a job change if the current job involves repetitive use of the hands. For other underlying causes, medical advice and true "detective work" may be necessary.

The majority of carpal tunnel sufferers have been found to have low levels of vitamin B_6. Various studies have shown that vitamin B_6 supplementation (usually at 5–100 milligrams per day for about three months) has relieved all symptoms in patients with low levels of vitamin B_6. But one should seek medical advice regarding long-term vitamin B_6 supplementation because it may cause nervous system disorders when used in doses as low as 200 milligrams daily over three years. There have been increasing numbers of vitamin B6-blocking substances in our environment. Blocking action can be caused by certain drugs, yellow dyes, and excessive protein intake. The drugs include isoniazid, hydralazine, dopamine, penicillamine, and oral contraceptives. (See INFLAMMATION in Part Two for more information.)

Dietary Modifications

1. Avoid all yellow dyes. Read labels.

2. Avoid excessive protein intake. The recommended daily allowance for protein is about 45 grams for women and 55 grams for men. One ounce of meat, chicken, or fish is equal to about 7 grams. In the starch category (which includes grains, corn, beans, and potatoes), one small potato, one-half cup of cereal, or one slice of bread yields about 3 grams of protein. To give you an example of how fast this adds up, consider one tuna sandwich to be about 20 grams of protein (one-half cup tuna contains 14 grams of protein; two slices bread contain 6 grams of protein). With one tuna sandwich, you have consumed almost half your protein needs for the day. Our recommendation is that you eat more vegetable sources of protein as found in beans, lentils, and split peas; whole grains; and fruit while reducing your intake of animal protein. If you wish to calculate your protein intake more accurately, you can purchase an inexpensive booklet from the American Diabetes Association titled *Exchange Lists for Meal Planning*, 1660 Duke St., Alexandria, VA 22314, or call (800) ADA-DISC.

Nutrients That Help

☐ **Vitamin B6** deficiency has been associated with carpal tunnel syndrome. Supplementation has shown relief of symptoms within a few weeks for many, with complete cure in eight to twelve weeks for about 85 percent of the patients. Others have benefited from the use of pyridoxal-5 phosphate or the addition of magnesium.

☐ **Bromelain** has excellent anti-inflammatory properties that have been shown to reduce swelling, bruising, pain, and healing time. It works best in combination with vitamin C.

☐ **Vitamin C** enhances the effects of bromelain.

☐ **Ginger** has been shown in studies to have anti-inflammatory properties.

Beneficial Juices

☐ Kale, spinach, turnip greens, and green pepper—sources of vitamin B6.

☐ Pineapple—the only source of the enzyme bromelain.

☐ Kale, parsley, green pepper, and broccoli—sources of vitamin C.

☐ Ginger—has anti-inflammatory properties.

Suggested Juicing Recipes / Carpal Tunnel Syndrome

Bromelain Special

¼ pineapple, with skin	*Push pineapple through hopper.*

Green Surprise

1 large kale leaf 2–3 green apples, seeded Lime twist for garnish	*Bunch up kale leaf and push through hopper with apples. Garnish with lime twist. The surprise is that you won't taste the kale!*

Maureen's Spicy Tonic

¼ pineapple, with skin ½ apple, seeded ¼-inch slice ginger root	*Push pineapple through hopper with apple and ginger.*

Garden Salad Special

3 broccoli flowerets   *Push broccoli and garlic*
1 garlic clove   *through hopper with carrots*
4–5 carrots or 2 tomatoes   *or tomatoes. Follow with*
2 stalks celery   *celery and green pepper.*
½ green pepper

Ginger Fizz

¼-inch slice ginger root   *Push ginger through hopper*
1 apple, seeded   *with apple. Pour juice into*
Sparkling water   *ice-filled glass. Fill glass to*
                              top with sparkling water.

Ginger Hopper

¼-inch slice ginger root   *Push ginger through hopper*
4–5 carrots, greens removed   *with carrots and apple.*
½ apple, seeded

CATARACTS

A cataract is a clouding or opacity of the lens of the eye or its capsule or both. It is characterized by a gradual loss of vision. Cataracts can be caused by eye diseases, surgery, injury, systemic diseases, exposure to ultraviolet light or radiation, toxins, hereditary disease, and the process of aging.

Cataracts form because of an inability to maintain normal concentrations of sodium, potassium, and calcium within the lens of the eye. It appears that the cellular pump that pumps out sodium and pumps in potassium becomes less efficient. This loss of efficiency is most often due to free-radical damage to a portion of the sulfur-containing proteins, enzymes, and cell membranes in the lens, which includes the sodium-potassium pump. Free-radical damage can come from exposure to ultraviolet rays and low levels of radiation from x-rays.

General Recommendations

It is possible to stop the progression of cataracts if they are treated during their early development. If you suspect that you have a cataract, contact an opthalmologist immediately. Diet can be an important adjunct to this treatment.

The herbal extract bilberry is rich in bioflavonoids and assists in removing chemicals from the eye's retina.

The Chinese herbal preparation hachimijiogan has been used to increase glutathione levels in the lens. It has been used in China and Japan to treat cataracts quite successfully.

Avoid bright light and direct eye contact with sunlight by wearing sunglasses whenever you are outdoors.

Dietary Modifications

1. Increase your consumption of legumes—beans, lentils, and split peas—which are high in sulfur-containing amino acids.

2. Consume generous portions of green, red, and yellow vegetables and fruits and their juices. These foods are high in vitamin C and carotenoids, like beta-carotene, all of which destroy free radicals.

3. Increase your consumption of seeds such as sunflower, nuts such as almonds, and whole grains, wheat germ, and wheat germ oil. These foods are excellent sources of vitamin E, a powerful antioxidant.

4. A folk remedy calls for drinking two ounces of green bean juice three times a day. (You'll need to mix this with milder-tasting juices such as carrot or tomato.)

5. Avoid foods that generate free radicals, including fried, smoked, and barbecued foods, as well as rancid foods.

6. A cleansing diet is recommended to help in ridding the body of heavy metals. (See the Cleansing Diets, page 299.)

This could be very therapeutic, since levels of heavy metals such as cadmium have been shown to be significantly higher in the lens of a cataract patient than they are in the normal lens.

Nutrients That Help

☐ **Beta-carotene** is an antioxidant that protects the eye lens from light-induced damage.

☐ **Vitamin B$_1$** is an important nutrient in intracellular eye metabolism.

☐ **Vitamin B$_2$** deficiency has been linked with cataracts. But once the cataract has formed, research shows that supplementation with vitamin B$_2$ can do more harm than good, since it interacts with light and oxygen to form superoxide radicals. No more than 10 milligrams of supplemental vitamin B$_2$ is recommended per day for a person with cataracts. (This does *not* include the vitamin B$_2$ contained in food.)

☐ **Vitamin C** is an antioxidant that has been shown to stop the progression of cataracts. It is known to lower intraocular pressure.

☐ **Vitamin E** is an antioxidant that protects the eyes from the damage of free radicals.

☐ **Selenium** is an antioxidant that helps prevent free-radical damage. A deficiency is associated with cataract formation.

☐ **Copper, manganese, and zinc** have been shown to be helpful in halting and reversing cataract growth.

☐ **Glutathione** is an enzyme and antioxidant that protects the lens from free-radical damage.

Beneficial Juices

☐ Carrot, kale, parsley, and spinach—sources of beta-carotene.

☐ Garlic—a "juicable" source of vitamin B$_1$.

☐ Spinach, currant, asparagus, broccoli, Brussels sprout—sources of vitamin B$_2$.

☐ Kale, parsley, green pepper, and broccoli—sources of vitamin C.

☐ Spinach, asparagus, and carrot—sources of vitamin E.

☐ Red Swiss chard, turnip, garlic, and orange—sources of selenium.

☐ Carrot, garlic, and ginger root—sources of copper.

☐ Spinach, turnip greens, beet greens, and carrot—sources of manganese.

☐ Ginger root, parsley, garlic, and carrot—sources of zinc.

Suggested Juicing Recipes / Cataracts

Eye Therapy Express

2 endive leaves
Handful parsley
4–5 carrots, greens removed
2 stalks celery

Bunch up endive and parsley, and push through hopper with carrots and celery.

Mineral Tonic

Handful parsley
2 turnip leaves
1 kale leaf
4–5 carrots, greens removed

Roll up parsley in turnip and kale leaves, and push through hopper with carrots.

Garden Salad Special

3 broccoli flowerets
1 garlic clove
4–5 carrots or 2 tomatoes
2 stalks celery
½ green pepper

Push broccoli and garlic through hopper with carrots or tomatoes. Follow with celery and green pepper.

Harvest Soup

2–3 garlic cloves
1 kale leaf
1 large tomato
2 stalks celery
1 collard leaf, chopped
1 Tbsp. croutons

Roll garlic in kale leaf, and push through hopper with tomato and celery. Place juice in saucepan, add chopped collards, and gently heat. Garnish with croutons.

Ginger Fizz

¼-inch slice ginger root
1 apple, seeded
Sparkling water

Push ginger through hopper with apple. Pour juice into ice-filled glass. Fill glass to top with sparkling water.

Ginger Hopper

¼-inch slice ginger root
4–5 carrots, greens removed
½ apple, seeded

Push ginger through hopper with carrots and apple.

CELLULITE

Cellulite is a cosmetic disorder characterized by the appearance of "orange peel skin"—bumps, lumps, pitting, and deformation of the skin. It affects primarily women. Some of the symptoms associated with cellulite are feelings of tightness, tenderness, and heaviness in the affected areas. The thighs are the prime area to be affected.

General Recommendations

The good news is that cellulite can be reversed significantly. The most obvious recommendation is weight loss. (See the Weight-Loss Diets on page 319.) Women who are slim and athletic have the least amount of cellulite. Weight loss should be gradual, however, especially in women over forty. Rapid weight loss in women in this age group could make the "orange peel skin" more pronounced. In addition, exercise is very important in reducing cellulite. Be sure to get aerobic exercise (walking is a good choice) at least five times a week for a minimum of thirty minutes each time.

Leslie and Sussanah Kenton, in their book *Raw Energy*, state that the detoxifying properties of raw foods offer the most effective approach to preventing and reversing cellulite. They cite a relationship between cellulite and body toxicity based on the research of two French physicians, Merus-Blatter and Laroche. These researchers found that constipation was more common in women with cellulite, as was poor lymphatic drainage—the inefficient elimination of wastes that accumulate in spaces between cells. Other researchers have found a correlation between this condition and poor circulation, poor liver function, and an underactive thyroid.

To improve circulation in the affected areas and help remove waste products, the European technique of skin brushing is very effective. Purchase a long-handled natural bristle brush, which can be found at most health food stores. The Kentons suggest brushing the surface of the skin starting with your feet and moving up your legs, both front and back, with firm, sweeping strokes. Then move up your body brushing your back, stomach (in circular motions), arms, and neck. Avoid the face. Regular skin brushing can greatly improve lymphatic drainage. This is very important, the Kentons remind us, because as waste materials become trapped by connective tissues, they create pockets of water, toxins, and fat, giving the skin its "peau d'orange" appearance. The English authors note that with lots of exercise, skin brushing, and raw foods, this lumpy, bumpy skin will slowly disappear. So don't give up after the first couple of months!

One more step to rid the body of cellulite involves the strengthening of capillary walls. This is where raw food plays an important part. Bioflavonoids, which are abundant in many fruits and vegetables, have been shown to strengthen capillary walls. As capillary walls are strengthened, blood plasma has less chance of seeping through them into spaces between cells. It is this seepage that encourages the formation of cellulite.

Several botanical medicines, such as Centella Asiatica and Aescin, have been shown to be very beneficial in treating cellulite. In addition, topical applications of certain salves and ointments, such as Cola Vera extract and Fucus Vesiculosis, have demonstrated impressive results.

Dietary Modifications

1. Modify the Basic Diet (see page 285) so that 50–75 percent of your diet is composed of raw foods and their juices. Generously include citrus fruits, leaving the white pithy part on the fruit for juicing or eating because it contains the highest concentration of bioflavonoids, which strengthen capillary walls.

2. For weight loss, see the Weight-Loss Diets (page 319).

3. A cleansing diet can be very helpful in ridding the body of toxic accumulations and eliminating old fluids stored in tissue spaces. (See the Cleansing Diets, page 299.)

4. Eat plenty of high-fiber foods like oat bran, whole grains, legumes (beans, split peas, and lentils), vegetables, and fruits. In addition, get ample amounts of fluid, all of which will help prevent constipation.

5. Increase your consumption of foods that cleanse and support the liver, including beets and artichoke leaves. (Artichoke leaves can't be juiced.) The spice turmeric has also been used historically to protect the liver, as has dandelion root. (Steep one-half teaspoon of dandelion root per cup of hot water.) Milk thistle has also been used for its role in enhancing liver function.

Nutrients That Help

☐ **Vitamin C** deficiency has been associated with fragile capillaries.

☐ **Bioflavonoids** work synergistically with vitamin C. In addition, deficiency is associated with capillary permeability.

☐ **Vitamin E** deficiency has been associated with capillary permeability.

Beneficial Juices

☐ Kale, parsley, green pepper, and spinach—sources of vitamin C.

☐ Orange, grapefruit, cantaloupe, broccoli, parsley, and cabbage—sources of bioflavonoids. (For a more complete list of the bioflavonoids, see AGING in Part Two.)

☐ Spinach, asparagus, and carrot—sources of vitamin E.

Suggested Juicing Recipes / Cellulite

Evening Regulator

2 apples, seeded 1 pear	*Alternate pushing apple and pear slices through hopper.*

Cherie's Cleansing Cocktail

¼-inch slice ginger root 1 beet ½ apple, seeded 4 carrots, greens removed	*Push ginger, beet, and apple through hopper with carrots.*

Body Cleanser

½ cucumber 1 beet ½ apple, seeded 4 carrots, greens removed	*Push cucumber, beet, and apple through hopper with carrots.*

Ginger Hopper

¼-inch slice ginger root 4–5 carrots, greens removed ½ apple, seeded	*Push ginger through hopper with carrots and apple.*

Garden Salad Special

---

3 broccoli flowerets
1 garlic clove
4–5 carrots or 2 tomatoes
2 stalks celery
½ green pepper

Push broccoli and garlic through hopper with carrots or tomatoes. Follow with celery and green pepper.

Bioflavonoid Special

---

3 oranges, peeled (leave
    white pithy part)

Push orange segments through hopper.

Berry Cantaloupe Shake

½ cantaloupe, with skin
5–6 strawberries

Push cantaloupe and strawberries through hopper.

Liver Mover

---

1 small beet
2–3 apples, seeded

Push beet and apples through hopper.

CHOLESTEROLEMIA (HIGH CHOLESTEROL)

Cholesterolemia is defined as excess cholesterol in the blood. But cholesterol per se is not a "bad guy." The largest percentage of total body cholesterol is manufactured by the liver and is a normal part of bile. It plays an important part in your body's metabolism, serving as a precursor of various hormones, such as sex hormones, and building cell membranes.

Elevated blood cholesterol is the primary contributor to heart disease. Cholesterol makes up a large part of those fatty deposits that accumulate in the arteries, clogging them and causing cerebrovascular and cardiac insufficiency. And did you know that cholesterol also makes up the principal portion of most gallstones? It is implicated, as well, in impotence, mental impairment, and high blood pressure. High blood cholesterol has also been correlated with colon polyps and cancer.

General Recommendations

One of the goals in lowering blood cholesterol is to raise HDL (high-density lipoprotein) levels. They're the good lipoproteins that cause "reverse transport" of cholesterol from cells back to the liver. The other goal is to increase the consumption of essential fatty acids. Several studies have shown that essential fatty acids lower serum cholesterol. When a deficiency of these fatty acids exists, the body tends to produce more cholesterol in an attempt to produce substances known as prostaglandins, because biosynthesis of prostaglandins is enhanced by cholesterol as well as by essential fatty acids and other components. Prostaglandins are so important that the body will keep producing more and more cholesterol just so it can get enough prostaglandins for its needs. Now, you're probably wondering why prostaglandins are so important. They are vasodilators (agents that cause relaxation of blood vessels), inhibitors of blood clots, inhibitors of cholesterol, and facilitators of many other functions associated with the prevention of heart disease. The following strategies should be of value to you in lowering cholesterol and preventing and treating heart disease.

- **Stop smoking.** Nonsmokers have higher HDL levels than smokers.

- **Exercise frequently.** Reports show that even moderate aerobic exercises such as brisk walking pursued consistently (three or four times a week for a minimum of thirty minutes each time) has lowered levels of LDL (the "bad guy" low-density lipoproteins) and raised levels of HDL.

● **Monitor your blood cholesterol frequently.** Generally, your cholesterol level should be below 200.

Dietary Modifications

1. *Increase your intake of linoleic acid.* Studies were done in Norway after World War II to find out why death from cardiovascular disease showed a sharp decline during the war. It was found that linoleic acid consumption was much higher during wartime. Researchers have also found that men need about three to five times the linoleic acid that women need. This might account for the higher incidence of male heart attacks. Linoleic acid is commonly found in vegetable oils. The most effective source is cold-pressed flaxseed oil that has been bottled under carbon dioxide in the cold and kept refrigerated to prevent rancidity. One tablespoon of flaxseed oil per day is often recommended by nutritionally oriented doctors.

2. *Increase your consumption of whole grains.* Whole grains are good sources of linoleic acid. The postwar study in Norway found that more whole wheat and whole rye were eaten during the period when cardiovascular disease sharply declined. Other whole grains, like brown rice, are also beneficial. In addition, rolled oats and oat bran are rich in soluble fibers and have a very favorable effect on cholesterol, while psyllium husks (2 tablespoons daily, mixed in water) have reduced cholesterol by 10 to 14 percent.

3. *Reduce your cholesterol intake.* No more than 300 milligrams per day is the current recommendation. One large egg yolk contains 274 milligrams; three ounces of shrimp, 128 milligrams; three ounces of beef, 80 milligrams; one ounce of cheddar, 30 milligrams; and one tablespoon of butter, 12 milligrams.

4. *Significantly lower your intake of foods high in saturated fat.* This is just as important as reducing your intake of cholesterol-rich foods. Saturated fat should represent only about 10 percent of your daily diet. Avoid fried foods, and keep in mind that many fast-food restaurants use beef tallow for cooking their French fries, chicken, fish, and hamburgers.

Beef fat contains high amounts of both saturated fat and cholesterol, and frying temperatures above 400°F produce toxic substances.

5. Avoid margarine and hydrogenated oils. Margarine contains a substance known as trans-fatty acid, which inhibits prostaglandin production. Instead, make Better Butter by softening one pound of butter in your blender, adding one cup of vegetable oil, blending, and refrigerating. Substitute expeller-pressed or cold-pressed vegetable oils for all your cooking needs. Standard-fare oils contain trans-fatty acids, which can raise blood cholesterol. Conversely, cold-pressed olive oil has been shown to help reduce blood cholesterol. Other cold-pressed (not heated above 110°F) or expeller-pressed (using mechanical pressure exclusively) oils are also good choices. Look for the words "cold-pressed" or "expeller-pressed" on the label.

6. Avoid nondairy coffee creamers. Most of these milk substitutes contain coconut oil, a very saturated vegetable fat, along with a large amount of sweetener. Soymilk is a much better choice, and soybeans have been found to lower cholesterol.

7. Avoid refined carbohydrates. Sugar, alcohol, and refined flour are known to inhibit prostaglandin production. Sweeteners like refined sugar and fructose have also been shown to raise blood cholesterol and triglycerides. Read all labels. Many sugars are advertised falsely. For example, fructose is often the main ingredient in well-advertised "sugar-free" frozen yogurts. Instead of sweets, try fresh fruit, frozen fruit pops, or a fresh fruit smoothie! Instead of an alcoholic drink at happy hour, try a fresh juice cocktail. And bake or buy whole grain products.

8. Reduce your intake of coffee. Studies show that with an increased consumption of coffee, the blood cholesterol level goes up. Black tea (not herbal) can have the same effect.

9. Avoid regular table salt, and use sea salt sparingly. Season your foods with herbs, spices, garlic, onions, and chili peppers, including cayenne. Garlic has been shown to reduce blood cholesterol, slow the development of plaque, and inhibit blood clotting. Hot peppers also have an anticlotting effect.

10. There's still plenty left to eat. Now, you're probably wondering what you *can* eat. Well, the good news is: Plenty! Get your taste buds ready for the delectable flavors of succulent fruits and crisp vegetables. Toss your salads with lots of sprouts, especially alfalfa sprouts, which have been shown to lower cholesterol. Feast your eyes on the tantalizing colors of orange, green, and red fruit and vegetable juices. The soluble fibers pectin and guar gum have greater choles- terol-lowering effects than the insoluble fibers like cellulose and lignin (though they should not be rejected). Apples, pears, peaches, oranges, and grapes are good sources of pectins. And here's more great news: Soluble fibers will be present in your juices.

11. Generously consume legumes. Beans (such as soybeans, pinto beans, and navy beans), split peas, and lentils are among the foods found to lower cholesterol.

12. Increase your consumption of omega-3 fatty acids. These "good fats," which must be supplied by the diet, are necessary for carrying fat-soluble vitamins like A, D, E, and K; for hormone synthesis; for skin function; and for cell wall synthesis. They also lower blood cholesterol and triglycerides and reduce the tendency of blood to clot. Fatty cold-water fish are among your best choices, and they include mackerel, herring, sardines, bluefish, salmon, tuna, Pacific oysters, and European anchovies. Cold-pressed flaxseed oil (buy only brands that are kept chilled in opaque bottles) is an excellent source of omega-3 fatty acids. Nut oils, safflower oil, and sunflower oil are also good sources, as are dark green vegetables.

13. Try the Juice Fast. The Juice Fast (see page 301) is one way to lower cholesterol. For example, carrot juice has been shown to flush fat from bile in the liver, helping to lower cholesterol.

14. Design a new diet plan. If you want to replace your diet of high-fat, high-cholesterol foods with a sensible eating plan that is designed for gradual changes (the kind shown most likely to last), we recommend *The New American Diet* by Sonja and William Connor. Their dietary changeover is designed to take place in three phases. One word of caution, however (and this is where we differ from other authors): A product that is low in fat (like imitation sour cream and margarine) is not necessarily healthful. A considerable number of manmade low-fat products can cause other health problems over the long term.

Nutrients That Help

☐ **B-complex vitamins** are necessary in fat metabolism and are protective for the liver. Vitamin B6 and niacin have been shown to increase production of prostaglandins. (*Warning:* Niacin tablet supplementation is not recommended without strict medical supervision because of its side effects.)

☐ **Vitamin C** deficiency is associated with elevated cholesterol levels. This vitamin is known to lower cholesterol, especially when combined with bioflavonoids. Vitamin C is also known to increase prostaglandin production.

☐ **Vitamin E** improves circulation.

☐ **Chromium** may reduce total cholesterol and triglycerides, and raise HDL cholesterol.

☐ **Copper** deficiency is associated with elevated cholesterol levels.

☐ **Magnesium** deficiency can cause spasms of the coronary arteries. Supplementation may reduce total cholesterol, raise HDL levels, and inhibit platelet aggregation (clumping).

☐ **Potassium** deficiency is associated with arrhythmia, a change in the normal pattern of the heart beat.

☐ **Selenium** may reduce platelet aggregation.

☐ **Zinc** is known to increase the production of prostaglandins.

☐ **Coenzyme Q10** improves circulation.

Beneficial Juices

☐ Carrot, apple, ginger root, orange, and strawberry—all have demonstrated the ability to lower LDL levels.

☐ Green leafy vegetables—sources of B-complex vitamins.

☐ Kale, parsley, and green pepper—sources of vitamin C.

☐ Grape, parsley, and lemon—sources of bioflavanoids. (*See* AGING in Part Two for a more complete list.)

☐ Spinach, asparagus, and carrot—sources of vitamin E.

☐ Potato, green pepper, apple, and spinach—sources of chromium.

☐ Carrot, garlic, and ginger root—sources of copper.

☐ Beet greens, spinach, parsley, and garlic—sources of magnesium.

☐ Parsley, garlic, spinach, and cantaloupe—sources of potassium.

☐ Red Swiss chard, garlic, and orange—sources of selenium.

☐ Ginger root, turnip, parsley, garlic, and carrot—sources of zinc.

☐ Spinach—source of coenzyme Q_{10}.

Suggested Juicing Recipes / Cholesterolemia

Garden Salad Special

3 broccoli flowerets
1 garlic clove
4–5 carrots or 2 tomatoes
2 stalks celery
½ green pepper

Push broccoli and garlic through hopper with carrots or tomatoes. Follow with celery and green pepper.

Ginger Hopper

¼-inch slice ginger root
4–5 carrots, greens removed
½ apple, seeded

*Push ginger through hopper
with carrots and apple.*

Potassium Broth

Handful parsley
Handful spinach
4–5 carrots, greens removed
2 stalks celery

*Bunch up parsley and
spinach leaves, and push
through hopper with carrots
and celery.*

Anti-Cholesterol Cocktail

Handful parsley
Handful spinach
1 garlic clove
4 carrots, greens removed
Dash Tabasco sauce

*Bunch up parsley and
spinach, and push through
hopper with garlic and
carrots. Add Tabasco.*

Sprout Salad Express

Handful spinach
Handful alfalfa sprouts
4–5 carrots, greens removed
1 apple, seeded

*Bunch up spinach and
sprouts, and push through
hopper with carrots and
apple.*

Monkey Shake

½ orange, peeled (leave
    white pithy part)
½ papaya, peeled
1 banana
Orange twist for garnish

*Push orange through hopper
with papaya. Place juice and
banana in blender or food
processor, and blend until
smooth. Garnish with orange
twist.*

Berry Cantaloupe Shake

½ cantaloupe, with skin
5–6 strawberries

Push cantaloupe and
strawberries through hopper.

Gingerberry Pops

1 quart blueberries
1-inch slice ginger root
1 medium bunch green
    grapes
3-oz. paper cups
Wooden popsicle sticks

Push blueberries and ginger
through hopper with grapes.
Pour juice into cups, add
sticks, and freeze.

Hawaiian Fizz

3 pineapple rings, with skin
¼-inch slice ginger root
½ pear
Sparkling water
Pineapple spear for garnish

Juice pineapple. Push ginger
through hopper with pear.
Pour juice into a tall glass
and fill with sparkling water.
Garnish with pineapple spear.

CHRONIC FATIGUE SYNDROME

Chronic fatigue syndrome is a mononucleosis-like syndrome of unknown cause. Some people believe it is caused by a chronic infection with Epstein-Barr virus (EBV), and many chronic fatigue sufferers do show an infection. Symptoms include long-term low-grade fever, headache, recurring sore throat, upper respiratory infections, fatigue, lymph node swelling, intestinal problems, muscle and joint pain, irritability and mood swings, anxiety, depression, temporary memory loss, and sleep disturbances.

General Recommendations

No cure for chronic fatigue syndrome exists, because no drug has been discovered that can kill the virus (when one is present) or eliminate the symptoms. But there is hope. Author Cherie and her husband John have both had chronic fatigue syndrome. John had EBV antibodies detectable in his blood. Neither has chronic fatigue syndrome today.

Healing involves a comprehensive approach that includes a variety of therapies. The goal is to strengthen the immune system and cleanse the body. A complete detoxification program is recommended that involves support for the liver and encouragement of lymphatic flow and blood flow to the spleen. There are a variety of botanical medicines that can be very helpful in this process. See the *Encyclopedia of Natural Medicine* by Michael Murray and Joseph Pizzorno for a complete list. For advice regarding a comprehensive care approach to chronic fatigue syndrome that includes the use of botanical medicines, consult a naturopathic doctor (N.D.).

Stress reduction can be very beneficial for this condition. Psychological and physiological stress can have a detrimental effect on the immune system, and stress can play a major role in the development and progress of chronic fatigue syndrome. Many techniques are available to reduce psychological stress, including counseling, relaxation techniques, psychotherapy, and biofeedback. Become a positive thinker. Learn to laugh at life's events. Negative thoughts can harm the immune system. Nutritional therapy can accomplish much to alleviate physiological stress, but unless the psychological stressors are dealt with, the healing process will be impaired. It is best to address both areas when seeking wellness.

Get plenty of rest while your body is regaining strength. Avoid strenuous exercise, but try walking several times a week. As you get stronger, you may be able to add exercises such as low-impact aerobics.

Get a stool and/or blood test for candidiasis, and follow the dietary plan in this book if you test positive. (*See* CANDIDIASIS in Part Two.) Candida overgrowth is fairly common in cases of chronic fatigue syndrome.

Dietary Modifications

1. *Follow the Immune Support Diet.* (See page 293.)

2. *Eliminate all sweeteners.* Sugars have been shown to depress the immune system. Be sure to watch for "hidden sweeteners," too, like those found in muffins, pancake batter, cornbread, salad dressings, sweet and sour sauces, flavored yogurts, "sugar-free" frozen yogurt (it's loaded with sweetener), and health food store treats. Even alternative sweeteners like carob, fruit juice concentrate, and brown rice syrup should be avoided until the immune system becomes strong and your symptoms are gone.

3. *Avoid all foods made with refined (white) flour.* To do so, you will have to give up sourdough bread, pasta (whole wheat is fine), and hamburger buns. Just keep thinking about how good you will feel in the not-too-distant future.

4. *Avoid all alcohol, coffee, and black tea*. Herbal teas are fine.

5. *Eliminate all junk food, like chips, crackers with "bad stuff" in them, hot dogs, hamburgers, and pizza.*

6. *Choose whole, unprocessed foods.*

7. *Consume generous amounts of garlic, onions, ginger, and shiitake mushrooms, all of which enhance immune functions.*

8. *Juices are very beneficial for this condition, especially the green drinks, which can be made with any dark green vegetables, wheatgrass, or sprouts.* Dilute green drinks with milder-tasting juices, such as carrot, tomato, and apple. Try the recipes at the end of this section. Make at least 50 to 75 percent of your diet raw foods, with about half being juices and the other half being raw fruits and vegetables prepared in salads and "munchies." "Live foods" help to build a strong immune system.

9. *Include foods high in omega-3 fatty acids, such as cold-water fish like mackerel, herring, sardines, bluefish, salmon, tuna, Pacific oysters, squid, and European anchovies.* Cold-pressed flaxseed oil (buy only oil that has been refrigerated in opaque bottles) is very high in omega-3 fatty acids. Take one tablespoon per day. (It tastes fishy because it's the omega-3 fatty acids that give fish its taste and smell, so mix it with juice or yogurt.) Also, black currant seed oil capsules (two per meal), high in gamma linoleic acid (GLA) and the essential fatty acids, have been shown to be helpful for this condition.

10. Schedule a Juice Fast or any other cleansing diet. (See page 299.) If you don't have several days to fast, do what you can, even if it's just for one day.

Nutrients That Help

☐ **Beta-carotene** enhances immunity and protects against toxins.

☐ **Vitamin C** has antiviral effects, supports adrenal function, and enhances immunity.

☐ **Pantothenic acid** supports adrenal function and is an antistress nutrient.

☐ **B-complex vitamins** increase energy levels.

☐ **Selenium** protects the immune system.

☐ **Zinc** enhances immune function and protects the liver.

☐ **Coenzyme Q10** enhances immune function. Sources include sardines, mackerel, and salmon.

☐ **Multiple vitamin and mineral supplements** should be . taken with the juices to help rebuild the immune system.

Beneficial Juices

☐ Carrot, kale, parsley, and spinach—sources of beta-carotene.

☐ Kale, parsley, green pepper, and broccoli—sources of vitamin C.

☐ Broccoli, cauliflower, and kale—sources of pantothenic acid.

☐ Greens—the best source of many B vitamins. (Some B vitamins, such as vitamin B_{12}, are found primarily in animal products.)

☐ Red Swiss chard, turnip, garlic, and orange—sources of selenium.

☐ Ginger root, parsley, potato, garlic, and carrot—sources of zinc.

Suggested Juicing Recipes / Chronic Fatigue Syndrome

Ginger Hopper

¼-inch slice ginger root 4–5 carrots, greens removed ½ apple, seeded	*Push ginger through hopper with carrots and apple.*

Sprout Salad Express

Handful spinach Handful alfalfa sprouts 4–5 carrots, greens removed 1 apple, seeded	*Bunch up spinach and push through hopper with sprouts, carrots, and apple.*

Garden Salad Special

3 broccoli flowerets 1 garlic clove 4–5 carrots or 2 tomatoes 2 stalks celery ½ green pepper	*Push broccoli and garlic through hopper with carrots or tomatoes. Follow with celery and green pepper.*

Cherie's Cleansing Cocktail

¼-inch slice ginger root 1 beet ½ apple, seeded 4 carrots, greens removed	*Push ginger, beet, and apple through hopper with carrots.*

Potassium Broth

Handful parsley
Handful spinach
4–5 carrots, greens removed
2 stalks celery

Bunch up parsley and spinach leaves, and push through hopper with carrots and celery.

Calcium-Rich Cocktail

3 kale leaves
Small handful parsley
4–5 carrots, greens removed
½ apple, seeded

Bunch up kale and parsley, and push through hopper with carrots and apple.

Very Veggie Cocktail

Handful wheatgrass
½ handful parsley
Handful watercress
4 carrots, greens removed
3 stalks celery
½ cup chopped fennel
½ apple, seeded

Bunch up wheatgrass, parsley, and watercress, and push through hopper with carrots, celery, fennel, and apple.

Wheatgrass Express

Handful wheatgrass
2 mint sprigs
3-inch slice pineapple, with
   skin

Bunch up wheatgrass and mint, and push through hopper with pineapple.

Ginger Fizz

¼-inch slice ginger root
1 apple, seeded
Sparkling water

Push ginger through hopper with apple. Pour juice into ice-filled glass. Fill glass to top with sparkling water.

Berry Cantaloupe Shake

½ cantaloupe, with skin   *Push cantaloupe and*
5–6 strawberries   *strawberries through hopper.*

CIRCULATION PROBLEMS

Sluggish circulation can be caused by a variety of problems such as atherosclerosis (narrowing of arteries due to fatty deposits), Buerger's disease (inflammation of veins and arteries in lower parts of the body characterized by tingling sensations in fingers and toes), Raynaud's disease (constriction and spasms of blood vessels in extremities), or varicose veins. If poor circulation continues, be sure to see your doctor. Cold hands and feet, experienced mainly by women and often attributed to poor circulation, may actually be due to low tissue iron stores. It is best to increase iron stores not through iron tablets, but through increased consumption of iron-rich foods and their juices.

General Recommendations

It is important to get plenty of exercise on a consistent basis. Make it your goal to engage in aerobic exercise four times a week for a minimum of thirty minutes each time. Walking is a great form of exercise. It will improve the flow of blood and help keep your arteries unclogged and supple. Massage is another way to improve your circulation. Several kinds of massage, such as Swedish massage, will improve blood and lymph flow. At home, you can give yourself a massage with a long-handled natural bristle brush or a loofah mitt. Start at your feet and work upward and inward toward your heart. This is very stimulating before a bath or shower. It is also important to maintain normal weight.

Dietary Modifications

1. *Follow the Basic Diet.* (See page 285.)

2. *Eat a high-fiber diet that includes an abundance of fruits, vegetables, whole grains, legumes (beans, lentils, and split peas), seeds, and nuts.*

3. *Avoid high-fat foods such as red meat and dairy products.*

4. *Eliminate refined foods, including white flour products and sugar.*

5. *Avoid stimulants, including coffee, black tea, colas, and tobacco.*

6. *Avoid alcohol.*

7. *Limit your intake of very spicy foods.*

8. *See also* ATHEROSCLEROSIS and VARICOSE VEINS in Part Two.

Nutrients That Help

☐ **B-complex vitamins** improve circulation.

☐ **Germanium** enhances oxygen transport to tissues.

☐ **Chlorophyll** improves circulation.

Beneficial Juices

☐ Greens—the best source of many B vitamins. (Some B vitamins, such as vitamin B_{12}, are found primarily in animal products.)

☐ Garlic and onion—sources of germanium.

☐ Greens—excellent sources of chlorophyll.

Suggested Juicing Recipes / Circulation Problems

Potassium Broth

Handful parsley
Handful spinach
4–5 carrots, greens removed
2 stalks celery

Bunch up parsley and spinach leaves, and push through hopper with carrots and celery.

Garden Salad Special

3 broccoli flowerets
1 garlic clove
4–5 carrots or 2 tomatoes
2 stalks celery
½ green pepper

Push broccoli and garlic through hopper with carrots or tomatoes. Follow with celery and green pepper.

Green Goddess

Handful spinach
3 collard leaves
4 carrots, greens removed
2 stalks celery
½ cucumber
1 apple, seeded

Bunch up spinach and collard leaves, and push through hopper with carrots, celery, cucumber, and apple.

Very Veggie Cocktail

Handful wheatgrass
½ handful parsley
Handful watercress
4 carrots, greens removed
3 stalks celery
½ cup chopped fennel
½ apple, seeded

Bunch up wheatgrass, parsley, and watercress, and push through hopper with carrots, celery, fennel, and apple.

Spring Tonic

Handful parsley
4 carrots, greens removed
1 garlic clove
2 stalks celery

Bunch up parsley and push through hopper with carrots, garlic, and celery.

COLITIS

Colitis is inflammation of the colon. It is categorized as either mucous colitis or ulcerative colitis. Symptoms of mucous colitis, also called irritable bowel syndrome and spastic colon, include sudden attacks of diarrhea and spastic, colicky pain, often followed by constipation. Gelatinous mucus and shreds of mucous membrane may be passed.

Ulcerative colitis is a severe form of colitis. With this condition, there is ulceration of the mucosa of the colon. Symptoms include passage of a watery, offensive stool with mucus and pus. Abdominal pain, tenderness, or colic can be experienced. These symptoms can be accompanied by intermittent or irregular fever. Hemorrhage and perforation may occur. Anemia may be present due to loss of blood, along with dehydration and electrolyte, mineral, and trace element loss due to diarrhea. This disease usually occurs in people under the age of forty or fifty, although it can occur at any age. Ulcerative colitis is very nutritionally debilitating, and the sufferer should always receive nutritional and medical care.

Causes of colitis include stress, poor dietary habits, autoimmunity disorders (in which the body produces an immunological response to itself), bacteria, or an allergy to certain foods. Lactose (found in dairy products), wheat, or gluten (contained in wheat, oats, rye, and barley) intolerances are common. A food allergy test may be advisable. (See ALLERGIES in Part Two.)

General Recommendations

Good nutrition is an important part of the treatment for colitis. For some people, this alone may facilitate improvement. The diet should provide adequate protein and calories, and a high amount of vitamins and minerals. Frequent small meals are recommended rather than the customary three meals per day. Periodic dietary restrictions designed to "rest" the bowel also speed the healing process. Stress reduction can play an important part in treatment as well. Make mealtimes as pleasant as possible, and try to eat slowly and to chew foods very well.

Dietary Modifications / Ulcerative Colitis

1. Drink plenty of liquids to prevent fluid and electrolyte imbalance. Mix fruit juices half and half with water, mineral water, or aloe vera juice. Aloe vera juice can be very healing for the mucosa of the intestines. Drinking one-half cup in the morning and before bedtime can be beneficial. Carrot, cabbage, and green juices can be very healing as well.

2. During an acute phase or for healing of ulcerative lesions, bowel rest can be very beneficial. Eliminate all solid foods. Liquid diets consisting of fresh fruit and vegetable juices, and soymilk or almond milk provide nutrients and fluid while giving the bowel a rest. These liquids can be used to make a smoothie with a banana or other fresh fruit and hypoallergenic protein powder to increase protein intake. Vegetable soups and steamed vegetables can be liquefied by putting them through a blender. Mashed potatoes can also be prepared by whipping potatoes with potato water or unflavored soymilk. Use no butter, milk, or sour cream. Well-cooked cream of brown rice cereal topped with soy or almond milk makes a good breakfast meal. This bland and primarily liquid diet should be followed for about two weeks. Cleansing enemas may be very helpful at this time.

3. As healing progresses for ulcerative colitis, a low-fiber, bland, high-protein, high-calorie diet should be eaten in about six small meals a day. The diet should exclude nuts, seeds, whole grains, legumes (beans, lentils, and split peas), and raw fruits and vegetables. An exception is well-cooked brown rice, which may be tolerated well. Fresh fruit and vegetable juices make an excellent nutrient-rich dietary addition at this time. Dairy products, red meat, sugar products, processed foods, refined foods, fried foods, coffee, and spices should be strictly avoided.

4. Eat a low-fat diet. If your doctor has diagnosed steatorrhea (fatty stools and fat malabsorption), cut fat intake in half. Steatorrhea can be a major factor in the diarrhea of colitis patients, with fatty acids producing a cathartic effect on the colon's mucosa. Medium-chain triglycerides (MCTs) may be helpful at this time, since MCTs are more efficiently absorbed. (MCTs may be purchased at most pharmacies.)

5. High-potency vitamin and mineral supplements are recommended. Deficiencies of the following nutrients have been reported in hospitalized patients with inflammatory bowel disease: vitamin A, vitamin C, zinc, and vitamin K. Pancreatic enzyme supplements can be helpful to aid digestion.

6. Avoid all foods that aggravate your condition.

Dietary Modifications / Mucous Colitis

1. Drink plenty of liquids to prevent fluid and electrolyte imbalance. Mix fruit juices half and half with water, mineral water, or aloe vera juice. Aloe vera juice can be very healing for the mucosa of the intestines. Drinking one-half cup in the morning and before bedtime can be beneficial. Carrot, cabbage, and green juices can be very healing as well.

2. For mucous colitis, a high-fiber diet is recommended. Oat bran; whole grains, including brown rice; legumes; and fresh fruits and vegetables should constitute a large portion of the diet, unless any of these items are found to be irritating. Steam vegetables if they are not tolerated well raw. Vegetable juices are usually tolerated well, and are very healing for the intestinal tract. Eat fresh fruit at the end of a meal, not on an empty stomach. Avoid dairy products, red meat, processed foods, refined foods such as white flour, fried foods, coffee, sugar products, and spices. Obtain calcium from green juice drinks (see recipes) and low-fat yogurt, which can be tolerated by many lactose-intolerant individuals.

3. Supplementation with Lactobacillus acidophilus may be beneficial for both mucous colitis and ulcerative co-

litis. You may need to take it for weeks or months to experience symptom relief.

4. *Beneficial herbs include wild yam, chamomile, goldenseal, red clover, and yarrow.* Also beneficial are pau d'arco tea, garlic, and papaya.

5. *See also* DIARRHEA in Part Two.

Nutrients That Help

☐ **Beta-carotene** (which the body converts to Vitamin A) is necessary for tissue repair.

☐ **Folic acid** is helpful, as folate absorption is decreased in ulcerative colitis.

☐ **Vitamin C** with bioflavonoids is needed for mucous membrane healing.

☐ **Vitamin E** promotes tissue repair.

☐ **Vitamin K** deficiency has been linked with ulcerative colitis.

☐ **Calcium** helps prevent colon cancer.

☐ **Magnesium** promotes relaxation of the muscles in the bowel walls.

☐ **Zinc** promotes wound healing.

Beneficial Juices

☐ Carrot, kale, parsley, and spinach—sources of beta-carotene.

☐ Spinach, kale, and beet greens—sources of folic acid.

☐ Kale, parsley, green pepper, and broccoli—sources of vitamin C.

☐ Parsley, cabbage, sweet pepper, and broccoli—sources of bioflavonoids.

☐ Spinach, asparagus, and carrot—sources of vitamin E.

☐ Broccoli, lettuce, cabbage, and spinach—sources of vitamin K.

□ Kale, parsley, beet greens, and broccoli—sources of calcium.

□ Beet greens, spinach, parsley, and garlic—sources of magnesium.

□ Ginger root, parsley, garlic, and carrot—sources of zinc.

Suggested Juicing Recipes / Colitis

Calcium-Rich Cocktail

3 kale leaves
Small handful parsley
4–5 carrots, greens removed
½ apple, seeded

Bunch up kale and parsley, and push through hopper with carrots and apple.

Iron-Rich Drink

3 beet tops
4–5 carrots, greens removed
½ green pepper
½ apple, seeded

Bunch up beet tops, and push through hopper with carrots, followed by green pepper and apple.

Folic Acid Special

2 kale leaves
Small handful parsley
Small handful spinach
4–5 carrots, greens removed

Bunch up kale, parsley, and spinach, and push through hopper with carrots.

Vegetable Express

2 lettuce leaves
1 small wedge cabbage
4–5 carrots, greens removed
3 broccoli flowerets
½ apple, seeded

Bunch up lettuce leaves, and push through hopper with cabbage, carrots, broccoli, and apple.

Carotene Cocktail

Handful parsley
Handful spinach
4–5 carrots, greens removed
½ apple, seeded

*Bunch up parsley and
spinach, and push through
hopper with carrots and
apple.*

COMMON COLD

A cold is a viral infection of the upper respiratory tract. It is very contagious, and incubation time is eighteen to forty-eight hours in length. Lasting immunity does not develop.

Cold symptoms include congestion of nasal passages with a watery discharge, sneezing, and headaches. A cold may also be accompanied by a dry sore throat, fever, body aches, fatigue, and chills.

General Recommendations

The most effective method of preventing a common cold is to strengthen the immune system. More than one or two colds a year signals weakened immunity. If frequent colds are experienced, it is advisable to be checked for food allergies. A poor diet, physiological and psychological stress, and drug use (including the use of alcohol and tobacco) can all weaken the immune system.

When a cold "catches" you, there are steps you can take to shorten the recovery time.

Get plenty of rest in bed. Jobs and other obligations often force us to neglect our body. But lack of rest can hinder the body's defense mechanisms and prolong infection. When you rest in bed, and especially when you sleep, powerful immune-strengthening substances are released, enhancing the potency of your immune functions.

Drink plenty of fluids. The mucous membranes lining the respiratory tract must be kept hydrated. When they become dry, they offer a desirable breeding ground for viruses. A moist respiratory tract repels viral infections. Use a vaporizer, facial mist spray, or facial steamer, and drink liquids throughout the day.

Take warm ginger baths. Cut off several slices of ginger root and float them in a tub of warm water. Soak for about twenty minutes, and have a cup of Ginger Tea while you relax in the bath. (See the Ginger Tea recipe at the end of this section.)

Take hot footbaths. Dissolve a tablespoon of mustard powder in a bucket of hot water, and soak your feet for approximately ten minutes. Wrap your head in a towel at this time to increase your body heat.

Use lavender oil and eucalyptus oil to clear your throat and nose. Put six to eight drops of lavender oil or eucalyptus oil in a large pan of boiling water and reduce heat to a simmer. Wrap your head in a towel and inhale. These oils can be purchased at health food stores and from herbalists. *Do not use this treatment during pregnancy.* Use only half this amount of oil for children, and do not use for infants.

Dietary Modifications

1. Follow the Immune Support Diet. (See page 293.)

2. Avoid all sweets. Even fructose, honey, and orange juice have too much sugar. Sugars depress the immune system, limiting its ability to kill bacteria and viruses. In addition, blood sugar and Vitamin C compete for entry into white blood cells. All fruit juices—except orange juice, which should be avoided—should be diluted with at least equal parts of water. Vegetable juices are more beneficial than fruit juices.

3. Increase your consumption of green juices, especially those high in vitamin C. Make homemade vegetable soups and broths. Drink herbal teas, especially ginger (see recipe), pau d'arco, slippery elm, and echinacea.

4. Consume generous amounts of cayenne pepper, watercress, onions, and garlic. A folk remedy calls for chopping one garlic clove into tiny pieces and swallowing the garlic with a glass of water before bedtime. Cherie has successfully used this remedy many times.

5. Take acidophilus or megadophilus to replace "friendly" intestinal bacteria.

6. Try a cleansing diet for several days. (See the Cleansing Diets on page 299.)

7. *See also* SORE THROAT in Part Two.

Nutrients That Help

☐ **Beta-carotene** supports immune function and heals the epithelial tissues that line the respiratory tract.

☐ **Vitamin C** has antiviral and antibacterial action. This nutrient can shorten the course of the common cold and has proven beneficial in prevention.

☐ **Bioflavonoids** act synergistically with vitamin C and have antibacterial action as well.

☐ **Zinc** has antiviral activity.

Beneficial Juices

☐ Carrot, kale, parsley, and spinach—sources of beta-carotene.

☐ Kale, parsley, green pepper, and watercress—sources of vitamin C.

☐ Tomato, parsley, apricot, and lemon—sources of bioflavonoids. (See AGING in Part Two for a more extensive list.)

☐ Ginger root, parsley, garlic, and carrot—sources of zinc.

Suggested Juicing Recipes / Common Cold

Spring Tonic

Handful parsley
4 carrots, greens removed
1 garlic clove
2 stalks celery

Bunch up parsley and push through hopper with carrots, garlic, and celery.

Gazpacho Express

4 tomatoes
½ cucumber
¼ green pepper
1 garlic clove
2 stalks celery
Dash Tabasco sauce

Push tomatoes, cucumber, green pepper, and garlic through hopper with celery. Add Tabasco sauce.

Harvest Soup

2–3 garlic cloves
1 kale leaf
1 large tomato
2 stalks celery
1 collard leaf, chopped
1 Tbsp. croutons

Roll garlic in kale leaf, and push through hopper with tomato and celery. Place juice in saucepan, add chopped collards, and gently heat. Garnish with croutons.

Low-Sugar Pop

1 apple, seeded
¼ lime
Sparkling water

Juice apple and lime. Pour juice into tall, ice-filled glass. Fill glass to top with sparkling water.

Maureen's Spicy Tonic

¼ pineapple, with skin
½ apple, seeded
¼-inch slice ginger root

Push pineapple through hopper with apple and ginger.

Ginger Tea

2-inch slice ginger root
¼ lemon
1 pint water
1 stick cinnamon, broken
4–5 cloves
Dash nutmeg or cardamom

Juice ginger and lemon. Place juice in saucepan, and add water, cinnamon, and cloves. Gently simmer. Add nutmeg or cardamom.

Ginger Fizz

¼-inch slice ginger root
1 apple, seeded
Sparkling water

Push ginger through hopper
with apple. Pour juice into
ice-filled glass. Fill glass to
top with sparkling water.

Cherie's Cleansing Cocktail

¼-inch slice ginger root
1 beet
½ apple, seeded
4 carrots, greens removed

Push ginger, beet, and apple
through hopper with carrots.

Ginger Hopper

¼-inch slice ginger root
4–5 carrots, greens removed
½ apple, seeded

Push ginger through hopper
with carrots and apple.

CONSTIPATION

Constipation occurs when there is infrequent defecation, difficulty passing stools, or unduly hard and dry stools. Frequency of bowel movements varies, and there is no professionally agreed-upon frequency. But most nutritionally oriented physicians suggest one to two bowel movements daily. When fecal matter remains in the colon too long, harmful substances from bowel bacteria can contribute to many ailments, including flatulence, cellulite, hernias, hemorrhoids, varicose veins, indigestion, obesity, diverticulitis, insomnia, halitosis, headaches, and colorectal cancer. Chronic constipation has been associated with a higher incidence of colon cancer as well.

Constipation can be caused by poor dietary habits, insufficient fluid intake, food sensitivities, a sedentary lifestyle, lack of exercise, pregnancy, advanced age, iron tablets, certain drugs, metabolic disorders, endocrine problems, obstructions, bowel diseases, psychogenic disorders, insecticide exposure, and overuse of laxatives.

General Recommendations

Two types of constipation have been identified: atonic (lazy bowel) and spastic (narrowing of the colon with small, ribbon-like stools). For atonic constipation, a high-fiber diet with increased fluid intake is recommended. Also, bowel retraining is needed after constipation has been eliminated. There are four rules to follow in the retraining process. First, don't suppress the urge to defecate. Second, schedule regular times to sit on the toilet each day. Third, exercise at least four times per week for a minimum of twenty minutes each time. Fourth, discontinue the regular use of laxatives and enemas. (Mineral oil is not recommended at any time, since it interferes with fat-soluble vitamins.) The best approach is to train bowels to function independently.

Spastic constipation can be caused by an obstruction. See your doctor to rule out such complications. A more common cause is nervousness or anxiety. Relaxation exercises and positive thoughts can be very helpful.

Dietary Modifications

1. Numerous studies have shown the benefits of a high-fiber diet in the prevention and treatment of constipation. Conversely, a low-fiber diet can cause constipation. Increase your consumption of fresh fruits and vegetables, legumes, whole grains, seeds, and nuts. Particularly effective are foods containing cellulose—grains, fruits, vegetables, and seeds—because of their bulking capacity. Bran is the most concentrated form of cellulose fiber. You can start by eating one tablespoon of bran per day, and gradually increase your intake to five or six tablespoons daily. But be aware! Too much bran can reduce your body's ability to absorb calcium, magnesium, iron, and zinc.

2. Avoid constipating foods and drinks, including cheese, fried foods, sweets, white flour, salt, junk food, beef, pasteurized milk, wine, carbonated drinks, and coffee.

3. For spastic constipation, it may be necessary to decrease fiber until the situation is corrected. In this case, fruit and vegetable juices are an excellent means of obtaining adequate nutrients.

4. Psyllium seed husks make a safe laxative. Mix one or two rounded teaspoons in a glass of water and take after meals. Prunes and prune juice contain a laxative substance found to stimulate intestinal movement. Apples also have a laxative effect.

5. Take Lactobacillus acidophilus or megadophilus to restore friendly bowel bacteria. Overuse of laxatives and enemas can remove the beneficial bacteria and contribute to chronic constipation.

6. Juice fasting for several days can be very beneficial. (See the Juice Fast, page 301.)

Nutrients That Help

☐ **Folic acid** is beneficial if a deficiency exists.

☐ **Thiamin (Vitamin B₁)** is beneficial if a deficiency exists.

Beneficial Juices

☐ Spinach, kale, beet greens, and cabbage—sources of folic acid.

☐ Garlic—contains appreciable amounts of thiamin. (Thiamin is found primarily in seeds, nuts, beans, and whole grains.)

☐ Prune, pear, and apple—have a laxative effect.

Suggested Juicing Recipes / Constipation

Evening Regulator

2 apples, seeded
1 pear

Alternate pushing apple and pear slices through hopper.

Alkaline Special

¼ head cabbage (red or
    green)
3 stalks celery

Push cabbage and celery through hopper.

Tropical Squeeze

1 firm papaya, peeled
¼-inch slice ginger root
1 pear

Juice papaya. Push ginger through hopper with pear.

Cherie's Cleansing Cocktail

¼-inch slice ginger root
1 beet
½ apple, seeded
4 carrots, greens removed

Push ginger, beet, and apple through hopper with carrots.

Spring Tonic

Handful parsley
4 carrots, greens removed
1 garlic clove
2 stalks celery

Bunch up parsley and push through hopper with carrots, garlic, and celery.

CRAMPS

See MENSTRUAL PROBLEMS; MUSCLE CRAMPS.

CRAVINGS

Have you ever found yourself wandering aimlessly through your kitchen in the evening, snacking on a little bit of everything you can think of, only to continue searching for that "magic something" that will satisfy your hidden hunger? How about the uncontrollable urge for chocolate chip cookies—the kind of craving that causes you to eat half the dough before you've baked the cookies? Most people have experienced such cravings, and most wish they would go away—forever. Webster defines "crave" as "to want greatly," and that fairly well sums up a food craving—wanting that bag of potato chips or the chocolate ice cream pie more urgently than you want cellulite-free thighs.

Cravings for really strange items like dirt, starch, or paint are referred to as "pica." This phenomenon has been recorded for centuries, and it has long been explained as a need for minerals. That's also the current explanation for most familiar cravings—a need for specific nutrients. Cravings can also be due to food allergies, candidiasis, or PMS. (Or else you're pregnant!)

General Recommendations

Getting rid of cravings means getting to the root cause of those strange food urges. It's recognizing that even though you are ravenously hungry for a whole quart of pistachio ice cream or both bags of pretzels, that isn't what your body needs biochemically. The chances are strong that it needs something very different. That's what you can explore in this section. Find what you crave and put into practice the recommendations for modifying your diet. And the next time you get one of those uncontrollable urges, reach for fruits and vegetables instead of junk food, and make a big glass of juice that will give your body something it really needs.

Dietary Modifications and Nutrients That Help

There are five common types of food cravings, each of which has its own causes requiring specific dietary modifications.

Cravings for Sweets and Chocolates

If you're a person who finds delight in the mere aroma of a chocolate bar or who salivates at the sight of an ice cream cone, help is near. Certain nutrients may help you lose your craving for sweets. Often a craving for sweets is caused by a deficiency of the mineral chromium. Try eating more foods rich in chromium, including brewer's yeast, whole wheat, oysters, potatoes, green pepper, chicken, and apples. You may temporarily need to supplement with chromium drops (two to three drops per day), the most beneficial being liquid, trivalent organic chromium. Evening primrose oil and vitamin E may also be helpful. If you are a vegetarian, especially a vegan, you may be protein-deficient, a condition that can also cause a craving for sweets. Make sure you are eating at least two bowls of legumes (beans, split peas, or lentils) daily, plus several servings of whole grains rich in protein, such as brown rice, millet, or quinoa.

Beneficial Juices

☐ Green pepper, apple, spinach, and carrot—sources of chromium.

☐ Spinach, asparagus, and carrot—sources of vitamin E.

Cravings for Salty Foods

If potato chips, pretzels, bacon, or popcorn is your desire, it may be the salt you're really after. Salt cravings can be a symptom of sickle cell anemia, various muscular disorders, high blood pressure, diabetes, or various other disorders. You may want to seek a doctor's advice to rule out any serious problem. The cause of occasional salt cravings is often adrenal stress, which can be the result of caffeine consumption or of other factors. Overstressed, weakened adrenal glands allow blood pressure and blood sugar levels to drop, bringing on fatigue. Increasing salt intake can temporarily help the symptoms, but can have negative long-term results. Consumption of regular table salt should be reduced, and organic potassium should be increased. In addition, pantothenic acid (which you may need to supplement), vitamin C, vitamin B6, magnesium, and zinc will help feed and support the adrenal glands.

Beneficial Juices

☐ Parsley, garlic, spinach, and carrot—sources of potassium.

☐ Broccoli, cauliflower, and kale—sources of pantothenic acid.

☐ Kale, parsley, green pepper, and spinach—sources of vitamin C.

☐ Kale, spinach, turnip greens, and sweet pepper—sources of vitamin B6.

☐ Beet greens, spinach, parsley, and garlic—sources of magnesium.

☐ Ginger root, parsley, potato, garlic, and carrot—sources of zinc.

Cravings for Ice (Pagophagia)

If you walk around with a glass of ice continually in hand, you may have pagophagia. A craving for ice is often a sign of anemia. Anemia can be the result of iron, vitamin B12, and/or folic acid deficiency. A blood test is advisable. Foods highest in iron include brewer's yeast, wheat bran, pumpkin seeds, sunflower seeds, millet, parsley, liver, clams, and almonds. Vitamin C increases the absorption of iron sevenfold. Include vitamin C-rich foods such as sweet peppers, kale, parsley, or broccoli with iron-rich foods. Liver, clams, oysters, sardines, eggs, trout, salmon, and tuna are high in vitamin B12. Folic acid-rich foods include brewer's yeast, black-eyed peas, rice germ, soy flour, wheat germ, liver, legumes, asparagus, walnuts, and spinach. In addition, include plenty of juice drinks that are high in nutrients you lack. (*See also* ANEMIA in Part Two.)

Beneficial Juices

☐ Parsley, beet greens, spinach, and broccoli—sources of iron.

☐ Kale, parsley, green pepper, broccoli, and spinach—sources of vitamin C.

☐ Spinach, kale, beet greens, and broccoli—sources of folic acid.

Cravings for Peanut Butter

Do you ever find yourself in the peanut butter jar scooping out spoonfuls without even bothering with bread or crackers? If you often reach for the peanut butter, this is probably a true craving. Beware! Peanut butter can contain a good deal of rancid oil, and when combined with copper (which peanuts are rich in), this can create powerful free radicals that damage your cells, causing aging and disease. Peanuts are also a plentiful source of aflatoxins, a highly carcinogenic mold. So it's important to shake the peanut butter habit.

Unless you buy the brands that contain only peanuts and salt, it may be the corn syrup or other sugars you're really addicted to. Read the section on sugar cravings. Or, it may be copper that your body actually needs. Choose other copper-rich foods, such as oysters, Brazil nuts, almonds, hazelnuts, walnuts, pecans, split peas, liver, buckwheat, and lamb. Make juice drinks high in copper as well (see recipes). Dr. Douglas Hunt, author of *No More Cravings*, has helped his peanut butter cravers with calcium lactate and kelp tablets, or niacinamide and Complex F. See *No More Cravings* for more information.

Beneficial Juices

☐ Carrot, garlic, ginger root, coconut, and apple—sources of copper.

Cravings for Sour Foods

If you crave lemons or other sour foods, your body may need acetic acid to help detoxify a chemical produced from decaying proteins. This chemical builds up in the body due to putrefying foods in the intestinal tract. Make sure you deal with constipation promptly. (*See* CONSTIPATION in Part Two.) If you do not suffer from constipation, try drinking one teaspoon of lemon juice in water to provide acetic acid. Foods that are rich in riboflavin (Vitamin B_2)—including brewer's yeast, liver, almonds, wheat germ, wild rice, mushrooms, eggs, millet, and wheat bran—have also proven beneficial, probably because they assist in acetic acid metabolism. Chlorophyll, which, of course, is abundant in green juices, can also be helpful in reducing cravings for sour foods.

Beneficial Juices

☐ Kale, parsley, broccoli, and beet greens—sources of riboflavin (vitamin B_2).

☐ Green vegetables—high in chlorophyll.

Suggested Juicing Recipes / Cravings

Sugar Cravings

Ginger Hopper

¼-inch slice ginger root
4–5 carrots, greens removed
½ apple, seeded

Push ginger through hopper with carrots and apple.

Popeye's Favorite

Small handful spinach
4–5 carrots, greens removed
½ apple, seeded

Bunch up spinach and push through hopper with carrots and apple.

Garden Salad Special

3 broccoli flowerets
1 garlic clove
4–5 carrots or 2 tomatoes
2 stalks celery
½ green pepper

Push broccoli and garlic through hopper with carrots or tomatoes. Follow with celery and green pepper.

Cherie's Cleansing Cocktail

¼-inch slice ginger root
1 beet
½ apple, seeded
4 carrots, greens removed

Push ginger, beet, and apple through hopper with carrots.

Mineral Tonic

Handful parsley
2 turnip leaves
1 kale leaf
4–5 carrots, greens removed

Roll up parsley in turnip and kale leaves, and push through hopper with carrots.

Salt Cravings

Potassium Broth

Handful parsley
Handful spinach
4–5 carrots, greens removed
2 stalks celery

Bunch up parsley and spinach leaves, and push through hopper with carrots and celery.

Garlic Express

Handful parsley
1 garlic clove
4–5 carrots, greens removed
2 stalks celery

Bunch up parsley and push through hopper with garlic, carrots, and celery.

Tomato Salad Express

Handful spinach
Handful parsley
2 tomatoes
½ green pepper
Dash Tabasco sauce

Bunch up spinach and parsley, and push through hopper with tomatoes and green pepper. Add Tabasco sauce.

Chlorophyll Cocktail

3 beet tops
Handful parsley
Handful spinach
4 carrots, greens removed
½ apple, seeded

Bunch up beet tops, parsley, and spinach, and push through hopper with carrots and apple.

Ice Cravings

Folic Acid Special

2 kale leaves
Small handful parsley
Small handful spinach
4–5 carrots, greens removed

Bunch up kale, parsley, and spinach, and push through hopper with carrots.

Iron-Rich Drink

3 beet tops
4–5 carrots, greens removed
½ green pepper
½ apple, seeded

Bunch up beet tops, and push through hopper with carrots, followed by green pepper and apple.

Spring Tonic

Handful parsley
4 carrots, greens removed
1 garlic clove
2 stalks celery

Bunch up parsley and push through hopper with carrots, garlic, and celery.

Popeye's Favorite

Small handful spinach
4–5 carrots, greens removed
½ apple, seeded

Bunch up spinach and push through hopper with carrots and apple.

Peanut Butter Cravings

Pineapple Cocktail

3-inch slice pineapple, with skin
½ apple, seeded
½ cup coconut milk

Push pineapple through hopper with apple. Pour juice into glass and add coconut milk.

Ginger Hopper

¼-inch slice ginger root
4–5 carrots, greens removed
½ apple, seeded

Push ginger through hopper with carrots and apple.

Garlic Express

Handful parsley
1 garlic clove
4–5 carrots, greens removed
2 stalks celery

Bunch up parsley and push through hopper with garlic, carrots, and celery.

Sour Foods Cravings

Chlorophyll Cocktail

3 beet tops
Handful parsley
Handful spinach
4 carrots, greens removed
½ apple, seeded

Bunch up beet tops, parsley, and spinach, and push through hopper with carrots and apple.

Calcium-Rich Cocktail

3 kale leaves
Small handful parsley
4–5 carrots, greens removed
½ apple, seeded

Bunch up kale and parsley,
and push through hopper
with carrots and apple.

Cherie's Famous Lemonade

3–4 apples, seeded
¼ lemon

Push apples and lemon
through hopper.

Christmas Cocktail

2 apples, seeded
1 large bunch grapes
1 lemon wedge

Push apples, grapes, and
lemon through hopper.

CROHN'S DISEASE

Crohn's disease is a chronic inflammatory bowel disease that usually develops in individuals who are between fifteen and thirty-five years of age. It is characterized by intermittent bouts of diarrhea, low-grade fever, anorexia, weight loss, abdominal tenderness, flatulence, and malaise. Causes of Crohn's disease include genetic predisposition, infectious agents, immunologic abnormalities, and dietary factors. If the disease continues for years, bowel function can deteriorate. With deterioration comes impaired absorption of nutrients, which can weaken the immune system and delay healing. This condition can also increase the risk of colon cancer.

General Recommendations

Avoid stress as much as possible. During attacks, rest. A heating pad may help relieve pain. Daily bowel movements are extremely important. Diet is of primary consideration.

Dietary Modifications

1. A high-fiber, high-complex carbohydrate diet has been shown to be very beneficial. Wheat bran may be too irritating, but most high-fiber foods should be tolerated well, including fruits, vegetables, whole grains, seeds, and nuts. Dietary fiber has a positive effect on intestinal flora.

2. For very active Crohn's disease, an elemental diet is an effective nontoxic alternative to corticosteroids. In an elemental diet, which is usually administered in a hospital, protein is provided through predigested or free form amino acids.

3. An elimination diet is highly recommended for chronic inflammatory bowel diseases. In an elimination diet, offending foods are identified and eliminated from the diet. (See page 296 for details.) The most common of these foods are wheat and dairy products. A rotation diet may also be beneficial. We recommend Sally Rockwell's *The Rotation Game.*

4. Avoid all products containing carrageenan, which is extracted from an edible seaweed. Carrageenan is added to milk products such as ice cream, cottage cheese, and milk chocolate for its ability to stabilize milk proteins. In studies, animals that were fed carrageenan solutions developed bloody diarrhea and ulcerative colitis.

5. Drink plenty of fluids such as purified water, fresh juices, and herbal teas.

6. Avoid fried, greasy, and high-fat foods, spicy foods, pepper, tobacco, caffeine, alcohol, dairy products, margarine, carbonated beverages, animal proteins (with the exception of white fish), and refined carbohydrates, especially sweets.

Nutrients That Help

☐ **Folic acid** may be deficient due to poor absorption or inadequate diet.

☐ **Vitamin A** may be deficient.

☐ **Vitamin B₁₂** may be deficient. Speak to your doctor about supplementation, as this nutrient cannot be obtained from juices.

☐ **Vitamin C** may be deficient.

☐ **Vitamin D** may be deficient. Speak to your doctor about supplementation, as this nutrient cannot be obtained from juices.

☐ **Vitamin K** may be deficient.

☐ **Calcium** may be deficient.

☐ **Magnesium** may be deficient.

☐ **Selenium** may be deficient

☐ **Zinc** may be deficient.

Beneficial Juices

☐ Spinach, kale, beet greens, and broccoli—sources of folic acid.

☐ Carrot, kale, parsley, and spinach—sources of beta-carotene, which the body converts into vitamin A.

☐ Kale, parsley, green pepper, and broccoli—sources of vitamin C.

☐ Turnip greens, broccoli, lettuce, and cabbage—sources of vitamin K.

☐ Parsley, watercress, beet greens, and broccoli—sources of calcium.

☐ Beet greens, spinach, parsley, and garlic—sources of magnesium.

☐ Red Swiss chard, garlic, and orange—sources of selenium.

☐ Ginger root, parsley, garlic, and carrot—sources of zinc.

Suggested Juicing Recipes / Crohn's Disease

Calcium-Rich Cocktail

3 kale leaves
Small handful parsley
4–5 carrots, greens removed
½ apple, seeded

*Bunch up kale and parsley,
and push through hopper
with carrots and apple.*

Digestive Special

Handful spinach
4–5 carrots, greens removed

*Bunch up spinach and push
through hopper with carrots.*

Potassium Broth

Handful parsley
Handful spinach
4–5 carrots, greens removed
2 stalks celery

*Bunch up parsley and
spinach leaves, and push
through hopper with carrots
and celery.*

Chlorophyll Cocktail

3 beet tops
Handful parsley
Handful spinach
4 carrots, greens removed
½ apple, seeded

*Bunch up beet tops, parsley,
and spinach, and push
through hopper with carrots
and apple.*

Harvest Soup

2–3 garlic cloves
1 kale leaf
1 large tomato
2 stalks celery
1 collard leaf, chopped
1 Tbsp. croutons

*Roll garlic in kale leaf, and
push through hopper with
tomato and celery. Place juice
in saucepan, add chopped
collards, and gently heat.
Garnish with croutons.*

Garlic Express

Handful parsley   Bunch up parsley and push
1 garlic clove   through hopper with garlic,
4–5 carrots, greens removed   carrots, and celery.
2 stalks celery

Ginger Fizz

¼-inch slice ginger root   Push ginger through hopper
1 apple, seeded   with apple. Pour juice into
Sparkling water   ice-filled glass. Fill glass to
                                     top with sparkling water.

CYSTITIS

See BLADDER INFECTION.

DEPRESSION

Depression is a mental state characterized by extreme feelings
of dejection, sadness, and emptiness. Symptoms can include
poor appetite accompanied by inadequate diet and weight loss,
or increased appetite with weight gain; insomnia or excess
sleep; changes in usual activities; loss of interest; fatigue; loss
of concentration; feelings of worthlessness or inappropriate
guilt; and thoughts of suicide or death. In certain cases,
depression is appropriate to a life event. To be diagnosed as
depression, the depressed state (including at least four of these
symptoms) must be experienced for at least one month and
should be defined as inappropriate to life's events. The causes
of depression are categorized as psychological, sociological,
biochemical, or physiological. Specifically, they can include an

overreaction to life's events or to stress, lack of sunlight during winter months (seasonal affective disorder), nutritional deficiencies, poor diet, sugar (read the book *Sugar Blues* by William Dufty), caffeine, nicotine, thyroid and adrenal gland disorders, hormonal imbalances, allergies, environmental and microbial factors, or any serious physical disorder.

General Recommendations

Studies have found that choline (an amine found in plant and animal tissues) levels are extremely high in depressed patients. An abnormality in choline transport may be involved in this disease. This is one instance in which biochemical imbalances may be the cause of depression. Good nutrition is a vital adjunct to appropriate psychiatric care. Studies have shown that nutrients can profoundly influence biochemistry and brain activity. Among nutritionally oriented doctors, it is believed that diet is often the cause of depression and that our Western diet—which emphasizes junk food, snacking, and poor eating habits—is the primary contributor. The brain's neurotransmitters, which regulate behavior, are controlled by the food we eat.

Exercise is also a valuable component of depression therapy. Exercise alone has effected tremendous improvements in mood and stress management. A current study has shown decreased depression with increased physical activity. So walk your dog. If you don't have one, rent a four-legged friend! Do whatever it takes to get yourself moving.

And laugh! The old adage "Laughter is the best medicine!" is as true today as when it was coined. Rent some funny movies. Look for humor in your day. Keep a positive outlook. Start smiling more. External behavior is eventually internalized.

For help in coping with food allergies, which can cause your depression, see *Allergy Recipes* and *The Rotation Game* by Sally Rockwell, or try the Elimination Diet. (See page 296.)

Dietary Modifications

1. Eat plenty of high-quality protein, found in fish, turkey, and legumes (beans, lentils, and split peas). Proteins containing essential fatty acids that increase alertness are recommended; these are found in salmon and white fish. Inadequate protein consumption may lower the body's levels of iron, thiamin, riboflavin, niacin, and vitamins B_6 and B_{12}; increase your intake of foods that contain these nutrients. Also increase consumption of calcium-rich foods, such as greens, corn tortillas with lime added, almonds, sunflower seeds, and low-fat yogurt. Emotional stress lowers levels of nitrogen (found in protein) and calcium.

2. If you are taking a monoamine oxidase-inhibiting antidepressant drug (such as Nardil, Marplan, and Parnate, among others), restrict tyramine-containing foods. These foods include aged cheese, beer, red wine, ale, pickled herring, chicken liver, broad bean pods, canned figs, sausage, salami, pepperoni, commercial gravies, ripe avocado, fermented soy sauce, ripe banana, yeast concentrates, and pickled or smoked fish. Spoiled, overripe, and aged products should also be avoided.

3. Avoid saturated fats. Fats can inhibit the synthesis of neurotransmitters in the brain in that they cause the blood cells to clump together, resulting in poor circulation to the brain.

4. Avoid caffeine and sugar. Research has indicated that some individuals experience a tremendous lift after eliminating the consumption of sweets. In addition, some individuals experience an improvement in mood after eliminating caffeine.

5. Increase your consumption of tryptophan-rich foods. Tryptophan is the amino acid essentially responsible for the production of serotonin, the brain substance responsible for mood elevation and normal sleep. The transport of tryptophan to the brain may be inhibited in depressed individuals. Tryptophan vies with other amino acids for entry into the brain, and other amino acids are usually in larger quantity in a protein-rich meal. But a carbohydrate-rich meal has been shown to help the body's ability to absorb tryptophan. An example of a good combination is a turkey sandwich on whole grain bread. Turkey is high in tryptophan, and whole grain bread supplies ample complex carbohydrates. Milk, bananas, figs, and dates are other sources of tryptophan.

6. Increase your consumption of raw fruits and vegetables and their juices, and of legumes and whole grains. These foods are high in complex carbohydrates, which can stimulate the production of brain serotonin.

7. Try a one- to five-day Juice Fast. (See page 301.) Cherie found that many of her nutrition clients reported an increased sense of well-being following the Juice Fast.

Nutrients That Help

☐ **Biotin** deficiency may cause depression. This nutrient is abundant in soybeans, whole wheat flour, and rice bran.

☐ **Folic acid** deficiency may cause depression.

☐ **Vitamin B6** deficiency can be caused by the use of monoamine oxidase-inhibiting antidepressants.

☐ **Riboflavin** deficiency has been associated with depression.

☐ **Thiamin** deficiency is common in depression.

☐ **Vitamin B12** deficiency may cause depression. See your doctor about supplementation.

☐ **Vitamin C** deficiency has been associated with depression.

☐ **Calcium** supplementation may be especially effective for the elderly and in postmenopausal and postpartal depressions.

☐ **Iron** deficiency has been associated with depression.

☐ **Magnesium** deficiency has been associated with depression.

☐ **Potassium** deficiency has been associated with depression.

☐ **Omega-6 fatty acids,** abundant in evening primrose oil, may be deficient in depression.

Beneficial Juices

☐ Spinach, kale, beet greens, and broccoli—sources of folic acid.

☐ Kale, spinach, turnip greens, and sweet pepper—sources of vitamin B6.

☐ Kale, parsley, broccoli, and beet greens—sources of riboflavin.

☐ Garlic—a source of thiamin.

☐ Kale, parsley, green pepper, and broccoli—sources of vitamin C.

☐ Kale, parsley, broccoli, and spinach—sources of calcium.

☐ Parsley, beet greens, dandelion greens, and spinach—sources of iron.

☐ Beet greens, spinach, parsley, and garlic—sources of magnesium.

☐ Parsley, garlic, spinach, and carrot—sources of potassium.

Suggested Juicing Recipes / Depression

Chlorophyll Cocktail

3 beet tops
Handful parsley
Handful spinach
4 carrots, greens removed
½ apple, seeded

Bunch up beet tops, parsley, and spinach, and push through hopper with carrots and apple.

Calcium-Rich Cocktail

3 kale leaves
Small handful parsley
4–5 carrots, greens removed
½ apple, seeded

Bunch up kale and parsley, and push through hopper with carrots and apple.

Potassium Broth

Handful parsley
Handful spinach
4–5 carrots, greens removed
2 stalks celery

Bunch up parsley and spinach leaves, and push through hopper with carrots and celery.

Garlic Express

Handful parsley
1 garlic clove
4–5 carrots, greens removed
2 stalks celery

*Bunch up parsley and push
through hopper with garlic,
carrots, and celery.*

Garden Salad Special

3 broccoli flowerets
1 garlic clove
4–5 carrots or 2 tomatoes
2 stalks celery
½ green pepper

*Push broccoli and garlic
through hopper with carrots
or tomatoes. Follow with
celery and green pepper.*

Green Surprise

1 large kale leaf
2–3 green apples, seeded
Lime twist for garnish

*Bunch up kale leaf and push
through hopper with apples.
Garnish with lime twist. The
surprise is that you won't
taste the kale!*

DIABETES MELLITUS

Diabetes mellitus is a chronic disorder of carbohydrate, fat, and protein metabolism, characterized by high levels of blood glucose. It results from insufficient production of insulin by the pancreas. Without insulin, the body cannot utilize glucose; this creates a high level of glucose in the blood. Diabetes is the number-three killer in the United States. Diabetes mellitus has been categorized into five groups: Type I, insulin-dependent diabetes mellitus (IDDM); Type II, non-insulin-dependent diabetes mellitus (NIDDM); Type III, secondary diabetes; Type IV, gestational diabetes; and Type V, impaired glucose tolerance.

Diabetes mellitus is strongly associated with our Western diet. It is not common in cultures eating a more "primitive" diet—a diet consisting of whole grains, vegetables, and fruits, with little or no animal proteins and no refined foods. Obesity is also strongly associated with diabetes mellitus, especially NIDDM.

Of the five types of diabetes mellitus, the first two types are the most common. Symptoms of diabetes mellitus Type I can include unusual thirst, fatigue, frequent urination, nausea or vomiting, and unusual hunger. Type I usually occurs in children or young adults, and is commonly treated with insulin injections and diet. Symptoms of Type II can include blurred vision, itching, unusual thirst, drowsiness, obesity, fatigue, skin infections, poor wound healing, and tingling or numbness in the feet. Type II usually develops later in life, and can most often be controlled with dietary changes.

General Recommendations

Exercise is very helpful in the diabetes treatment plan. Many benefits have been observed, including enhanced insulin sensitivity, with a diminished need for insulin injections; improved glucose tolerance; increased numbers of insulin receptors; reduced serum cholesterol and triglycerides with increased HDL levels; and improved weight loss in obese diabetics. The physical fitness program must be carefully planned for the diabetic, however, to avoid risks.

Diet may be the most important factor in the treatment of diabetes. James Anderson popularized the high-carbohydrate plant-fiber diet (HCF, or High-Carbohydrate Fiber), which has received considerable support and substantiation in scientific literature as the diet of choice for this disorder. The diet recommended by the American Diabetes Association and the American Dietetic Association, utilizing the exchange lists, is considered by many nutritionally oriented doctors and nutritionists to be inferior to the HCF diet. The exchange diet is much higher in protein, cholesterol, and fat than the HCF diet. The exchange diet is based on six food groups—milk, vegetables, fruit, bread, meat, and fat. It allows 35 percent of the total calories as fat, an amount that has been shown to contribute to atherosclerosis. The carbohydrate content is much lower than that of the HCF diet, with 40–45 percent of total calories being derived from carbohydrates. Scientific studies have shown that a high-complex carbohydrate diet improves blood glucose control. The HCF diet consists of 70–75 percent complex carbohydrates (vegetables, fruit, legumes, and whole grains); 15–20 percent protein; and only 5–10 percent fat. We recommend the modified HCF (MHCF) diet over the HCF diet, because it contains restricted processed grains and excludes fruit juices, low-fiber fruits, skim milk, and margarine. The MHCF diet is described under "Dietary Modifications," below.

Dietary Modifications

1. *Follow a vegetarian or modified vegetarian diet (fish and poultry once a week).* This diet has been shown to reduce the risk of death from diabetes.

2. *Consume generous amounts of garlic and onions.* These foods have demonstrated significant blood sugar-lowering action.

3. *Consume generous amounts of raw foods and raw vegetable juices.* These foods have been found to be highly beneficial for diabetics. Dr. John Douglas discovered that raw high-fiber carbohydrates are better tolerated by diabetics than cooked ones, and that they help to stabilize blood sugar levels. These raw foods were found also to diminish cravings for more food. Dr. Max Bircher-Benner, founder of the famous European Bircher-Benner clinic, used raw juices as the pivot of many of his dietary treatments, including treatments for diabetic patients.

4. *Avoid fruit juices.* A few slices of apple used for sweetening a vegetable juice recipe may be tolerated, but if even this amount of fruit sugar is found to elevate blood glucose levels, it should not be used.

5. *Eliminate all sugars.* Sucrose has been associated with impaired glucose tolerance. All simple sugars (sweeteners) are eliminated on the HCF and MHCF diets. Sucrose and fructose have been shown to increase total serum cholesterol, LDL, triglyceride, and uric acid levels. We do not recommend artificial sweeteners as a substitute for sugar because of the health risks that have been linked with them.

Nutrients That Help

☐ **Vitamin B6** deficiency has been associated with diabetes.

☐ **Vitamin C** deficiency may exist.

☐ **Vitamin E** appears to be needed in increased amounts in diabetics.

☐ **Chromium** is a necessary component of the glucose tolerance factor. Glucose intolerance is one of the signs of chromium deficiency.

☐ **Copper** deficiency has been associated with glucose intolerance.

☐ **Magnesium** levels have been found to be significantly lower in diabetics.

☐ **Manganese** is needed for glucose metabolism.

☐ **Potassium** improves insulin sensitivity, responsiveness, and secretion.

☐ **Zinc** deficiency may play a role in the development of diabetes.

Beneficial Juices

☐ Kale, spinach, turnip greens, and sweet pepper—sources of vitamin B6.

☐ Kale, parsley, green pepper, and broccoli—sources of vitamin C.

☐ Spinach, asparagus, and carrot—sources of vitamin E.

☐ Potato, green pepper, apple, and spinach—sources of chromium.

☐ Carrot, garlic, and ginger root—sources of copper.

☐ Beet greens, spinach, parsley, and garlic—sources of magnesium.

☐ Spinach, beet greens, carrot, and broccoli—sources of manganese.

☐ Parsley, Swiss chard, garlic, and spinach—sources of potassium.

☐ Ginger root, parsley, potato, garlic, and carrot—sources of zinc.

Suggested Juicing Recipes / Diabetes Mellitus

Digestive Special

Handful spinach
4–5 carrots, greens removed

Bunch up spinach and push through hopper with carrots.

Potassium Broth

Handful parsley
Handful spinach
4–5 carrots, greens removed
2 stalks celery

Bunch up parsley and spinach leaves, and push through hopper with carrots and celery.

Chlorophyll Cocktail

3 beet tops
Handful parsley
Handful spinach
4 carrots, greens removed
½ apple, seeded

Bunch up beet tops, parsley, and spinach, and push through hopper with carrots and apple.

Garden Salad Special

3 broccoli flowerets
1 garlic clove
4–5 carrots or 2 tomatoes
2 stalks celery
½ green pepper

Push broccoli and garlic through hopper with carrots or tomatoes. Follow with celery and green pepper.

Tomato Salad Express

Handful spinach
Handful parsley
2 tomatoes
½ green pepper
Dash Tabasco sauce

Bunch up spinach and parsley, and push through hopper with tomatoes and green pepper. Add Tabasco sauce.

Garlic Express

Handful parsley
1 garlic clove
4–5 carrots, greens removed
2 stalks celery

Bunch up parsley and push through hopper with garlic, carrots, and celery.

Calcium-Rich Cocktail

3 kale leaves
Small handful parsley
4–5 carrots, greens removed
½ apple, seeded

Bunch up kale and parsley, and push through hopper with carrots and apple.

Low-Sugar Pop

1 apple, seeded
¼ lime
Sparkling water

Juice apple and lime. Pour juice into tall, ice-filled glass. Fill glass to top with sparkling water.

Pancreas Tonic

3 lettuce leaves
4–5 carrots, greens removed
Handful green beans
2 Brussels sprouts

Bunch up lettuce leaves and push through hopper with carrots, green beans, and Brussels sprouts.

DIARRHEA

Diarrhea is characterized by frequent, watery bowel movements. Other symptoms can include cramping and abdominal pain. Most commonly a symptom of gastrointestinal disturbances, diarrhea can also indicate more serious disorders such as dysentery, ulcerative colitis, or Crohn's disease. Diarrhea can be categorized as functional (due to stress or irritation); organic (due to intestinal lesion); osmotic (due to fat, lactose, simple carbohydrate, or gluten intolerances; artificial sweeteners; or excessive vitamin C intake); or secretory (due to viruses, bacteria, bile, acids, hormones, or laxatives). Secretory diarrhea is the most serious. Chronic diarrhea has been shown to be a common symptom of food allergies.

General Recommendations

Over-the-counter medications to stop diarrhea are not recommended. Your body may be ridding itself of toxic substances. If there is blood in the stool, the stools appear like black tar, or the situation persists for more than two or three days, see your doctor. If you experience chronic diarrhea (frequent recurrences), we recommend testing for food allergies. The Elimination Diet (see page 296) or the rotation diet (see *The Rotation Game* by Sally Rockwell) may be helpful.

Dietary Modifications

1. Drink plenty of fluids to prevent dehydration. Dehydration is characterized by a dry mouth and/or wrinkled skin. Replace electrolytes (minerals) with fresh juices. Fruit juices should be diluted with water. Carrot and green juices contain abundant minerals that make good electrolyte replacers. A long-used naturopathic remedy is to sip equal parts of sauerkraut and tomato juice. Cabbage juice may be substituted for sauerkraut juice, as substances in cabbage have been shown to heal intestinal lesions.

2. Avoid coffee (which can aggravate diarrhea), alcohol, and carbonated beverages, as well as all cold foods and drinks. Digestion is assisted by warmth. Rice water is beneficial and can be prepared by boiling one-half cup brown rice in three cups of water for forty-five minutes. Strain and drink three cups daily. Herbal teas such as chamomile, raspberry leaf, or blackberry leaf are helpful as well. Ginger Tea is useful for cramps and abdominal pain (see the recipes at the end of this section).

3. While experiencing diarrhea, it is advisable to avoid dairy products (except for plain yogurt), beans, fats, wheat, or any food suspected to be allergenic, as well as all solid foods. This is an appropriate time for a short Juice Fast. (See page 301.) Remember, though, to drink mostly vegetable juices.

4. As a supplement, try pectin, a soluble fiber that has long been a natural remedy for diarrhea. Pectin forms a gel-like substance when mixed in water. Try one tablespoon three times a day.

5. Take Lactobacillus acidophilus to restore friendly bacteria in the bowel. One-half teaspoon of acidophilus or megadophilus is suggested three times a day.

6. Follow the BRAT diet (banana, rice, apple, and tea), a traditional remedy for upset stomach and diarrhea.

7. As stools begin forming, reintroduce foods in small amounts. Soups, well-cooked brown rice, cream of brown rice cereal, plain yogurt, steamed vegetables, and grated apples make good choices.

8. *See also* COLITIS and INDIGESTION in Part Two.

Nutrients That Help

☐ **Folic acid** supplementation may be helpful for chronic diarrhea.

☐ **Sodium** can be lost in large quantities with diarrhea.

☐ **Potassium** can be lost in large quantities with diarrhea.

☐ **Magnesium** can be lost in large quantities with diarrhea.

☐ **Vitamin and mineral supplementation** may be needed to replace lost nutrients.

Beneficial Juices

☐ Spinach, kale, beet greens, and broccoli—sources of folic acid.

☐ Beet greens, beet, spinach, celery, and carrot—sources of organic sodium.

☐ Parsley, garlic, spinach, carrot, and red cabbage—sources of potassium.

☐ Beet greens, spinach, parsley, and beet—sources of magnesium.

Suggested Juicing Recipes / Diarrhea

Cabbage Cocktail	
¼ head cabbage 2 tomatoes	*Push cabbage and tomatoes through hopper.*

Digestive Special	
Handful spinach 4–5 carrots, greens removed	*Bunch up spinach and push through hopper with carrots.*

Ginger Tea	
2-inch slice ginger root ¼ lemon 1 pint water 1 stick cinnamon, broken 4–5 cloves Dash nutmeg or cardamom	*Juice ginger and lemon. Place juice in saucepan, and add water, cinnamon, and cloves. Gently simmer. Add nutmeg or cardamom.*

Garden Salad Special

3 broccoli flowerets
1 garlic clove
4–5 carrots or 2 tomatoes
2 stalks celery
½ green pepper

*Push broccoli and garlic
through hopper with carrots
or tomatoes. Follow with
celery and green pepper.*

Potassium Broth

Handful parsley
Handful spinach
4–5 carrots, greens removed
2 stalks celery

*Bunch up parsley and
spinach leaves, and push
through hopper with carrots
and celery.*

Spring Tonic

Handful parsley
4 carrots, greens removed
1 garlic clove
2 stalks celery

*Bunch up parsley and push
through hopper with carrots,
garlic, and celery.*

Veggie Cocktail

Handful parsley
3 beet tops
2 stalks celery
4 carrots, greens removed

*Bunch up parsley and beet
tops, and push through
hopper with celery and
carrots.*

DIVERTICULITIS

Diverticulitis is the inflammation of one or more sacs or pouches (diverticula) in the walls of the intestinal tract, causing a stagnation of feces in the distended sacs. Some patients experience no symptoms, but most complain of abdominal distention, cramps, elevated temperature, tenderness, diarrhea, or constipation. This is a disease that worsens with age and is due in part to the loss of tensile strength of intestinal mucosa. Poor diet and lack of exercise are the primary factors causing diverticular disease. Low-fiber, low-bulk diets contribute very little volume to the feces. Small-weight stools can cause a smaller bowel contraction, which produces obstruction. The pressure needed to push a dry, hard stool through the bowel can cause a diverticular "blow-out," resulting in the formation of pouches.

General Recommendations

Stretching exercises can be beneficial, and massaging the painful side can relieve discomfort. Enemas can help ease pain and rid the bowel of undigested and trapped foods. However, dietary changes are probably the most effective treatment for this disease.

Dietary Modifications

1. Eat a high-fiber diet. The old diet therapy for this disorder recommended low-roughage foods, but new research indicates that patients with diverticular disease who are placed on a high-fiber diet have less pain, defecate more easily, and experience less distention. The high-fiber diet consists of unprocessed bran, brown rice, whole grain cereals and breads, fruits, and vegetables.

2. During an acute phase, follow a Juice Fast (see page 301) or a modified fast. Carrot, cabbage, and green juices are very beneficial. You may also drink puréed vegetable soups.

3. Completely avoid nuts, seeds, dairy products (except plain yogurt), red meat, fried foods, spices, sweets, and processed foods.

4. Take pectin, psyllium seed husks, guar gum, or oat bran (fiber supplements) and acidophilus ("friendly" bowel bacteria) in the morning before breakfast.

Nutrients That Help

☐ **Beta-carotene** has a healing effect on the intestinal mucosa.

☐ **Vitamin K** deficiency has been linked to intestinal disorders.

Beneficial Juices

☐ Carrot, kale, parsley, and spinach—sources of beta-carotene.

☐ Turnip greens, broccoli, lettuce, and cabbage—sources of vitamin K.

Suggested Juicing Recipes / Diverticulitis

Lettuce Salad

3 lettuce leaves
3 carrots, greens removed
2 stalks celery
½ apple, seeded

Bunch up lettuce and push through hopper with carrots, celery, and apple.

Alkaline Cocktail

¼ head cabbage
3 ribs celery
3 carrots, greens removed

Push cabbage, celery, and carrots through hopper.

Harvest Soup

2–3 garlic cloves
1 kale leaf
1 large tomato
2 stalks celery
1 collard leaf, chopped
1 Tbsp. croutons

Roll garlic in kale leaf, and push through hopper with tomato and celery. Place juice in saucepan, add chopped collards, and gently heat. Garnish with croutons.

Cabbage Cocktail

¼ head cabbage
2 tomatoes

Push cabbage and tomatoes through hopper.

Digestive Special

Handful spinach
4–5 carrots, greens removed

Bunch up spinach and push through hopper with carrots.

Spring Tonic

Handful parsley
4 carrots, greens removed
1 garlic clove
2 stalks celery

Bunch up parsley and push through hopper with carrots, garlic, and celery.

EATING DISORDERS

See OVERWEIGHT/OBESITY; UNDERWEIGHT.

ECZEMA (ATOPIC DERMATITIS)

This condition has become synonymous with chronic dermatitis. In early stages, the skin may be itchy, red, and swollen, with small blisters and a weeping of fluids. Later, the skin generally becomes crusted, scaly, and thickened. Other possible symptoms include burning, the appearance of papules, and a tendency for the skin to become overgrown with bacteria. Studies have shown that eczema is, at least partially, an allergic response. Low stomach acid (hypochlorhydria) has been associated with both eczema and food allergies. Stress can also contribute to eczema.

General Recommendations

The control of food allergies is a very important part of eczema control. If you suspect that you are allergic to certain foods but are unsure as to which ones, ask your doctor for a food allergy screening test. Skin-scratch tests are not always efficient means of determining food allergies; the RAST or ELISA blood test is recommended by many nutritionally oriented doctors. You may also try the Elimination Diet (see page 296), which will help identify those foods that may be causing problems.

Dietary Modifications

1. Increase you consumption of fatty cold-water fish such as mackerel, herring, sardines, bluefish, salmon, tuna, Pacific oysters, European anchovies, and squid. Patients with eczema have shown a deficiency or defect in essential fatty acid metabolism. This defect appears to result in a decreased production of anti-inflammatory substances. Studies have found that increasing the consumption of essential fatty acids by eating fatty fish at least twice a week and supplementing with fish oils, flaxseed oil (expeller- or cold-pressed), or evening primrose oil relieves symptoms of eczema. At the same time, the consumption of animal fats should be reduced, as these fats produce substances that are sources of inflammatory agents.

2. Increase your consumption of oats, as they have been found to have anti-inflammatory properties that are very helpful for eczema. Both raw and cooked oats are effective. Also, an oatmeal facial pack may be beneficial. (Mix one-half cup oats with water or a little yogurt, making a paste, and spread over face or other areas affected by eczema. Let dry for about fifteen minutes. Rinse well, and keep affected tissues dry and clean.) If there is any sign of infection, see your doctor. Don't attempt to treat infections yourself.

3. Use the Elimination Diet to identify food allergies. (See page 296.)

Nutrients That Help

☐ **Beta-carotene** deficiency can leave skin vulnerable to thickening, as found in eczema.

☐ **Bioflavonoids** are beneficial in controlling inflammation and allergy.

☐ **Selenium** may be deficient.

☐ **Zinc** supplementation may be beneficial.

Beneficial Juices

☐ Carrot, kale, parsley, and spinach—sources of beta-carotene, which is converted to vitamin A as needed.

☐ Parsley, cabbage, sweet pepper, and tomato—sources of bioflavonoids.

☐ Red Swiss chard, turnip, garlic, and orange—sources of selenium.

☐ Ginger root, parsley, potato, garlic, and carrot—sources of zinc.

☐ Cucumber—traditionally used to soothe the skin.

Suggested Juicing Recipes / Eczema

Beauty Spa Express

Small handful parsley
Handful spinach
4–5 carrots, greens removed
½ apple, seeded

Bunch up parsley and spinach, and push through hopper with carrots and apple.

Fresh Complexion Express

2 slices pineapple, with skin
½ cucumber
½ apple, seeded

Push pineapple through hopper with cucumber and apple.

Cucumber Cooler

1 tomato	*Juice tomato, pour juice into*
1 cucumber	*ice cube tray, and freeze.*
2 stalks celery	*Juice cucumber and celery.*
Parsley sprig for garnish	*Pour juice into tall glass, add*
	tomato cubes, and garnish
	with sprig of parsley.

Digestive Special

Handful spinach	*Bunch up spinach and push*
4–5 carrots, greens removed	*through hopper with carrots.*

Potassium Broth

Handful parsley	*Bunch up parsley and*
Handful spinach	*spinach leaves, and push*
4–5 carrots, greens removed	*through hopper with carrots*
2 stalks celery	*and celery.*

Garden Salad Special

3 broccoli flowerets	*Push broccoli and garlic*
1 garlic clove	*through hopper with carrots*
4–5 carrots or 2 tomatoes	*or tomatoes. Follow with*
2 stalks celery	*celery and green pepper.*
½ green pepper	

Ginger Hopper

¼-inch slice ginger root	*Push ginger through hopper*
4–5 carrots, greens removed	*with carrots and apple.*
½ apple, seeded	

EDEMA

See WATER RETENTION.

EPILEPSY AND SEIZURES

Epilepsy is a chronic disease characterized by seizures or attacks in which there can be loss of consciousness with a succession of convulsions. Some patients have frequent attacks occurring daily, while others have long periods of a year or two between episodes. Many children diagnosed with epilepsy outgrow their seizures and become seizure-free after the removal of medication.

Seizures vary in severity. A petit mal seizure, which is relatively mild, begins with a sudden loss of consciousness. Muscles may twitch or may lose tone. In a grand mal seizure, which is more extreme, the person will fall to the ground, lose consciousness, and have convulsions.

There are many forms of epilepsy, each characterized by specific symptoms. There are also many possible causes of epilepsy, including a variety of lesions of the central nervous system, food sensitivities, heavy metal toxicity, head injuries, hypoglycemia, or malnutrition, to name a few possibilities. All types of epilepsy, regardless of cause, involve an uncontrolled electrical discharge from brain nerve cells. This disorder affects approximately one percent of the United States population.

General Recommendations

Several studies have shown that identification of food sensitivities and appropriate dietary changes have effectively controlled or significantly reduced seizures. A food allergy test (ELISA or RAST blood tests are recommended) may be very helpful in controlling this condition. Or, try the Elimination Diet. (See page 296.)

Try to engage in consistent exercise, as this will improve circulation to the brain. Also try to minimize stress and tension as much as possible. Be aware that antiseizure medications often have side effects, including liver problems, memory impairment, and fatigue. Work with your doctor to keep drug doses as low as possible while following a diet to control seizures.

Dietary Modifications

1. *Follow the Basic Diet.* (See page 285.) Meals should be small, well balanced, and eaten at regular intervals. Avoid the consumption of large amounts of foods or fluids at one time. Small nutritious snacks can be eaten between meals.

2. *Avoid the consumption of aspartame (NutraSweet) and other artificial sweeteners, alcoholic beverages, caffeine, nicotine, sugar, and refined foods.*

3. *Reduce your consumption of animal proteins.*

4. *Each day, drink several glasses of juice made from green vegetables like kale, beet tops, leafy lettuce, chard, peas, and green beans.* These can be added to milder-tasting juices, like carrot or tomato juice.

Nutrients That Help

☐ **Folic acid** supplementation may be beneficial.

☐ **Vitamin B6** supplementation may be beneficial.

☐ **Magnesium** may suppress epileptic episodes.

☐ **Manganese** may be deficient.

☐ **Zinc** may be deficient. Anticonvulsants may cause zinc deficiency.

☐ **Choline** supplementation may be beneficial.

☐ **Taurine** (an amino acid) supplementation may be beneficial.

Beneficial Juices

☐ Spinach, kale, beet greens, and broccoli—sources of folic acid.

☐ Kale, spinach, sweet pepper, and potato—sources of vitamin B6.

☐ Beet greens, spinach, parsley, and garlic—sources of magnesium.

☐ Spinach, turnip greens, beet greens, and carrot—sources of manganese.

☐ Ginger root, turnip, parsley, garlic, and carrot—sources of zinc.

☐ Green pea, potato, green bean, and cabbage—sources of choline.

Suggested Juicing Recipes / Epilepsy

Seven-Vegetable Cocktail

2 kale leaves
2 beet tops
Handful spinach
3–4 carrots, greens removed
1 stalk celery
1 small garlic clove
1 scallion
½ cup cabbage

Bunch up kale, beet tops, and spinach. Push through hopper with carrots, celery, garlic, scallion, and cabbage.

Garden Salad Special

3 broccoli flowerets
1 garlic clove
4–5 carrots or 2 tomatoes
2 stalks celery
½ green pepper

Push broccoli and garlic through hopper with carrots or tomatoes. Follow with celery and green pepper.

Potassium Broth

Handful parsley
Handful spinach
4–5 carrots, greens removed
2 stalks celery

Bunch up parsley and spinach leaves, and push through hopper with carrots and celery.

Alkaline Special

¼ head cabbage (red or green)
3 stalks celery

Push cabbage and celery through hopper.

Ginger Hopper

¼-inch slice ginger root
4–5 carrots, greens removed
½ apple, seeded

Push ginger through hopper with carrots and apple.

EPSTEIN-BARR VIRUS

See CHRONIC FATIGUE SYNDROME.

EYE PROBLEMS

See CATARACTS.

FATIGUE

See CHRONIC FATIGUE SYNDROME.

FIBROCYSTIC BREAST DISEASE

See PREMENSTRUAL SYNDROME.

FOOD ALLERGIES

See ALLERGIES.

GAS

See COLITIS; INDIGESTION.

GINGIVITIS

See PERIODONTAL DISEASE.

GOUT

Often called the rich man's disease, gout is one of the oldest conditions recorded in medical history. This disorder occurs when the body produces excess uric acid and/or is unable to eliminate uric acid. This excess uric acid is the end product of the metabolism of purine, a compound that is present in many foods, primarily those of animal origin. The result is a blood level of uric acid that is three to fifteen times the normal level. The excess uric acid crystalizes in the joints and in other tissues, acting as an abrasive and causing swelling and intense pain, usually in the first joint of the big toe. Fever and chills may also be present. The first attack often occurs in the night, usually after an overconsumption of alcohol or purine-rich foods, trauma, the use of certain drugs, or surgery.

General Recommendations

Achieve and maintain a body weight 10 to 15 percent below ideal weight. Weight loss should not be drastic, but should be consistent over a period of months. A sudden reduction in calories can precipitate an acute attack of gout. For this reason, strict water fasts should be avoided. Also, because stress may precipitate an attack, you should seek means of stress reduction and relaxation. Most important is a diet that excludes purine-rich foods.

Dietary Modifications

1. Eliminate foods high in purines, which include meats, organ meats, gravies, shellfish, herring, sardines, mackerel, anchovies, and yeast. Foods containing moderate amounts of purine—fish, poultry, legumes, asparagus, mushrooms, and spinach—should be consumed in small portions only (one 2- to 3-ounce serving of fish or fowl, or 1/2 cup of one of the purine-containing vegetables per day). A diet restricted in purines will significantly reduce serum uric acid levels. A large portion of dietary protein should come from dairy products, eggs, vegetables, and whole grains.

2. Avoid all alcohol. Ethanol increases uric acid production. (Studies of patients with gout have shown that many patients consume above-average amounts of alcohol.)

3: Restrict fat intake. Fats are believed to reduce the normal excretion of uric acid.

4. Increase your consumption of complex carbohydrates. Try to eat at least 100 grams per day by boosting your intake of whole grains like brown rice, millet (high in protein), oats, popcorn, and vegetables. A high complex-carbohydrate diet increases the excretion of uric acid.

5. Avoid fructose, which increases uric acid production. Limit your intake of fruit juices.

6. Consume generous amounts of fluids to keep urine diluted. Drink a minimum of six to eight 8-ounce glasses of water per day. Also, include three or four glasses of vegetable juices per day (minimizing the vegetables that are high in purines, as noted above).

7. *Try the old folk remedy that calls for the consumption of one small dish of sour cherries every day for three weeks.* Research has confirmed that consuming one-half pound of fresh or canned cherries per day is effective in lowering the levels of uric acid and preventing attacks of gout.

8. *Decrease the inflammatory response by consuming a 3-ounce serving of fatty cold-water fish.* Fatty cold-water fish, like salmon and tuna, are high in omega-3 fatty acids, which have been shown to reduce the incidence of inflammatory disorders. (For more information, see INFLAMMATION in Part Two.)

Nutrients That Help

☐ **Folic acid** is said to reduce uric acid production.

☐ **Vitamin C** may lower serum uric acid by increasing excretion. Megadoses of supplemental vitamin C are not recommended, however, as they may increase uric acid levels in a small number of individuals.

☐ **Bromelain**, the enzyme in pineapple, is an effective anti-inflammatory agent.

☐ **Omega-3 fatty acids** may reduce inflammation.

Beneficial Juices

☐ Kale, beet greens, and broccoli—sources of folic acid.

☐ Kale, parsley, sweet pepper, and strawberry—sources of vitamin C.

☐ Pineapple—the only source of bromelain.

☐ Green vegetables—sources of omega-3 fatty acids.

☐ Cherry and strawberry—help neutralize uric acid.

Suggested Juicing Recipes / Gout

Cherry Cocktail

4 handfuls cherries, pitted
½ cup strawberries

Push cherries and strawberries through hopper.

Green Surprise

1 large kale leaf
2–3 green apples, seeded
Lime twist for garnish

Bunch up kale leaf and push through hopper with apples. Garnish with lime twist. The surprise is that you won't taste the kale!

Wheatgrass Express

Handful wheatgrass
2 mint sprigs
3-inch slice pineapple, with
   skin

Bunch up wheatgrass and mint, and push through hopper with pineapple.

Waldorf Salad

1 green apple, seeded
1 stalk celery

Push apple and celery through hopper.

Berry Cantaloupe Shake

½ cantaloupe, with skin
5–6 strawberries

Push cantaloupe and strawberries through hopper.

Strawberry Apple Delight

1–2 apples, seeded
6 strawberries

Push apple and strawberries through hopper. Garnish with strawberry.

Chlorophyll Cocktail

3 beet tops
Handful parsley
Handful spinach
4 carrots, greens removed
½ apple, seeded

*Bunch up beet tops, parsley,
and spinach, and push
through hopper with carrots
and apple.*

GUM DISEASE

See PERIODONTAL DISEASE.

HAIR LOSS (ALOPECIA)

Alopecia is natural or abnormal baldness or thinning of the hair. It can appear in patches or over the entire head. Hair loss can result from the aging process, surgery, radiation, severe illness, drugs, endocrine disorders such as hypothyroidism, sudden loss of weight, vitamin or mineral deficiency (especially iron), overconsumption of supplements such as vitamin A and niacin, poor diet, stress, certain forms of dermatitis, pregnancy, and hereditary factors. There are over a dozen types of alopecia. Therefore, if you suddenly lose large amounts of hair, it may be appropriate to consult your physician to rule out any underlying medical problem that may be causing this loss. Be aware, though, that it is normal to lose about forty to eighty hairs per day.

General Recommendations

Some people lose hair after an illness because of an accumulation of oils, dead cells, and medication residues at the hair follicle. These residues can "choke" the hair, causing it to fall out. Ask your beautician or beauty supply store about products that remove such residues from hair and scalp. A rinse of sage tea or apple cider vinegar can help hair grow, as can a scalp massage with ginger root juice tonic or with a tonic that combines cayenne pepper with vodka (see the tonic recipes at the end of this section). Lying on a slant board for fifteen to twenty minutes per day will cause blood to flow to the scalp, and daily scalp massages will also help improve circulation. To encourage hair growth, make an infusion with the herbs horsetail, catnip, and southernwood, and use as a rinse. Use only natural hair products; avoid using harsh chemical products on your hair.

Stimulating hair growth from within by the foods you eat is even more important than what you put on your scalp and hair. Vitamins, minerals, amino acids, and other nutrients provide the raw materials from which hair is produced. Our American diet is too rich in foods that actually "starve" the hair, such as fat, sugar, and refined foods. You may need to make certain dietary modifications to encourage your hair to grow.

Dietary Modifications

1. Follow the Basic Diet. (See page 285.)

2. Include plenty of foods rich in the sulfur-containing amino acids L-cysteine and L-methionine, which are found in animal products (eggs are an especially rich source), legumes, and cabbage. Skin, hair, and nails contain some of the body's most rigid proteins, all of which have a high sulfur content. Eat animal proteins in moderation, however. An ample serving of lean meat, poultry, or fish is three to five ounces, depending upon your body size. Eastern medicine says that eating too much meat can cause hair loss. This just might be true!

3. Cut down on sweets. Eastern medicine also says that too much sugar—especially fruit sugar (fructose)—can cause balding on the sides of the forehead. In her own practice, Cherie has found that sugar is often a contributing factor in hair loss, and that after sugar is removed from the diets of certain individuals, the hair-loss process is either halted or totally or partially reversed.

4. Include foods rich in the B vitamins, with special emphasis on choline, inositol, and PABA. Choline is plentiful in eggs, wheat germ, legumes (beans, split peas, and lentils), oatmeal, and brown rice. Lecithin, wheat germ, rice bran, whole wheat, and legumes are excellent sources of inositol. PABA is found in mushrooms, cabbage, sunflower seeds, wheat germ, oats, spinach, and eggs.

5. Make sure that your diet contains ample essential fatty acids. Eat fish two or three times a week (not deep-fried). If your hair is dry and brittle, you may improve its texture by supplementing your diet with primrose oil or pure cold- or expeller-pressed flaxseed oil (buy it only in refrigerated opaque bottles).

Nutrients That Help

☐ **B-complex vitamins** are essential for health and growth of hair.

☐ **Vitamin C** helps improve circulation to the scalp.

☐ **Vitamin E** improves hair health and enhances hair growth.

Beneficial Juices

☐ Green leafy vegetables—sources of B-complex vitamins.

☐ Kale, parsley, green pepper, and broccoli—sources of vitamin C.

☐ Spinach, asparagus, and carrot—sources of vitamin E.

☐ Alfalfa—helps to stimulate hair growth.

☐ Ginger juice—used traditionally to stimulate circulation to the scalp.

Suggested Juicing Recipes / Hair Loss

Hair-Growth Cocktail

---

2 dark green lettuce leaves
Handful alfalfa sprouts
4–5 carrots, greens removed

*Bunch up lettuce and alfalfa,
and push through hopper
with carrots.*

Very Veggie Cocktail

Handful wheatgrass
½ handful parsley
Handful watercress
4 carrots, greens removed
3 stalks celery
½ cup chopped fennel
½ apple, seeded

*Bunch up wheatgrass,
parsley, and watercress, and
push through hopper with
carrots, celery, fennel, and
apple.*

Ginger Hopper

¼-inch slice ginger root
4–5 carrots, greens removed
½ apple, seeded

*Push ginger through hopper
with carrots and apple.*

Potassium Broth

Handful parsley
Handful spinach
4–5 carrots, greens removed
2 stalks celery

*Bunch up parsley and
spinach leaves, and push
through hopper with carrots
and celery.*

Green Surprise

---

1 large kale leaf
2–3 green apples, seeded
Lime twist for garnish

*Bunch up kale leaf and push
through hopper with apples.
Garnish with lime twist. The
surprise is that you won't
taste the kale!*

Hair Growth Tonics

Ginger Juice Tonic

1- to 2-inch piece ginger root

Juice ginger root. Pour the juice on your head and massage into the scalp. Let dry for 10–15 minutes; then shampoo. Ginger root juice has been used naturopathically to stimulate circulation to the scalp. Your head will feel a tingling sensation, as if it just had a Certs!

Cayenne Pepper Tonic

4 oz. red cayenne pepper
1 pint 100-proof vodka

Mix red cayenne pepper with vodka. Let sit for two weeks, shaking the mixture several times. Then strain until the liquid is pepper free. (A nylon stocking works well for straining.) This makes liquid capsicum pepper. (This is not for drinking!) Each day, apply this mixture to thinning or bald areas of the scalp. Within five or six weeks, hair should begin to grow. (This may not work for hereditary baldness.)

HEADACHE

See MIGRAINE HEADACHE.

HEARTBURN

See INDIGESTION.

HEMORRHOIDS

See VARICOSE VEINS.

HERPES SIMPLEX I and II

Herpes simplex is a viral infection causing clusters of small blisters. Type I is usually found on the upper body. Most commonly, it is seen as a cold sore on the lips. Type II is usually found on the lower part of the body, and is commonly known as genital herpes. Genital herpes is sexually transmitted and is the most prevalent herpes infection. After entering the body, the virus never leaves, although it may lie dormant for long periods of time. During outbreaks, painful blisters form around the mouth and genitals. These blisters are highly infectious until healed. Genital herpes can cause serious complications during pregnancy. A pregnant woman who has had an outbreak of Type II at any time in the past should make the infection known to her doctor. There is no known way of killing this virus, so present treatment focuses on reducing the frequency and severity of outbreaks.

General Recommendations

This is definitely a case of "prevention is the best medicine." Avoid any direct contact with herpes blisters. An adult with a cold sore who kisses a child on the lips can give that child a lifelong viral infection! Once the original infection has healed, stimuli such as sunburn, stress, or food allergy can reactivate the virus. Stress reduction techniques may be helpful. Vitamin E applied as an oil to the blisters can reduce healing time.

Dietary Modifications

1. Follow the Immune Support Diet (see page 293), modifying it as described below.

2. Eat generous portions of all seafood, chicken, turkey, eggs, organ meats, potatoes, brewer's yeast, and dairy products (if tolerated). These foods are high in lysine, an amino acid that retards the growth of the herpes virus. Your consumption of these foods should be high at all times, and should be further increased during outbreaks. You might also ask your physician about supplementing your diet with lysine as a free-form amino acid.

3. During active outbreaks, avoid eating whole grains and whole grain products (cereals, breads, pasta, and pancakes); legumes (soybeans and soy products, lentils, peas, etc.); corn; sprouts; and foods containing seeds (eggplant, tomatoes, squash, etc.). The above foods should be eliminated during outbreaks because they contain approximately equal amounts of lysine, which retards viral growth, and the amino acid arginine, which appears to be necessary for the herpes virus to replicate. Between outbreaks, these foods may be eaten in moderation when balanced with lysine-rich foods and/or lysine supplements.

4. At all times, avoid the consumption of chocolate; nuts (peanuts, almonds, Brazil nuts, cashews, filberts, pecans, walnuts, etc.); nut butters; sugar, cakes, and other sweets; alcohol; coffee and tea; seed meal (tahini and sesame butter); sunflower seeds; coconut; and white flour foods. Some of these foods—for instance, the chocolate and nuts—should be avoided because they are high in arginine. The other foods—including sugar, alcohol, coffee, tea, and white flour products—inhibit immune system response.

Nutrients That Help

☐ **Beta-carotene** increases the action of interferon, a substance that your body uses to stop viruses from reproducing. It also stimulates the white blood cells to kill more viruses.

☐ **Vitamin C and bioflavonoids** compose another group of immune system strengtheners.

☐ **Zinc** inhibits viral replication and enhances the immune system.

□ **Polyphenols**, which are anutrients, inactivate viruses in the test tube and may do the same in your body.

□ **Lysine**, an amino acid, retards the growth of the herpes virus. Ask your doctor about lysine supplementation.

Beneficial Juices

□ Cantaloupe, carrot, and kale—excellent sources of beta-carotene.

□ Citrus fruit (with white pithy part intact)—sources of the vitamin C/bioflavonoid complex.

□ Ginger, carrot, and parsley—sources of zinc.

□ Apple, grape, and blueberry—good sources of polyphenols.

Suggested Juicing Recipes / Herpes Simplex I and II

Very Berry Virus Chaser

1 large bunch green grapes
1 large bunch red grapes
1 quart blueberries or
    blackberries

Juice green grapes. Pour juice into ice cube tray and freeze. Push red grapes and berries through hopper, and pour juice into tall glass. Add frozen grape cubes and garnish with small cluster of grapes.

Gingerberry Pops

1 quart blueberries
1-inch slice ginger root
1 medium bunch green
    grapes
3-oz. paper cups
Wooden popsicle sticks

Push blueberries and ginger through hopper with grapes. Pour juice into cups, add sticks, and freeze.

Applemint Fizz

4–6 sprigs fresh mint
2 green apples, seeded
1 small lemon wedge
Sparkling water
Mint sprig for garnish

Bunch up mint and push through hopper with apples and lemon. Juice directly into a small pitcher filled with ice. Pour juice into tall glass and fill with sparkling water. Garnish with sprig of mint.

Fruit Tea

1 orange, peeled (leave white pithy part)
1 red apple, seeded
1 lime wedge
1 quart water

Juice fruit. Place juice in saucepan, add water, and gently heat.

Veggie Cocktail

Handful parsley
3 beet tops
2 stalks celery
4 carrots, greens removed

Bunch up parsley and beet tops, and push through hopper with celery and carrots.

High-Calcium Drink

3 kale leaves
Small handful parsley
4–5 carrots, greens removed

Bunch up kale and parsley, and push through hopper with carrots.

HIGH BLOOD PRESSURE

See HYPERTENSION.

HIGH CHOLESTEROL

See CHOLESTEROLEMIA.

HYPERTENSION
(HIGH BLOOD PRESSURE)

Hypertension, also called high blood pressure, is defined as a repeatable blood pressure reading of greater than 150/90. In more than 90 percent of the people with hypertension, the disorder has no identifiable cause, although its risk is increased by excess weight, a high sodium level in the diet, a high cholesterol level, and a family history of high blood pressure. For some people, dietary changes can lower blood pressure. However, recent research shows that a dietary modification that lowers blood pressure in one individual may not have the same effect in another individual. Some detective work may be necessary, but the payoff could be your life. Hypertension is associated with an increased risk of heart disease and death. In past years it was common to prescribe drugs to lower blood pressure, but questions about the safety of this treatment are making diet and lifestyle changes much more attractive for some patients.

General Recommendations

Incorporate a regular form of exercise into your schedule. Walking is a good way to start. Eliminate smoking, and eliminate or greatly reduce alcohol and caffeine consumption. Stress reduction techniques such as biofeedback and yoga may be helpful for some people. If you are overweight, lose those extra pounds. Weight reduction consistently lowers blood pressure in overweight individuals.

Dietary Modifications

1. Follow the Basic Diet. (See page 285.)

2. Reduce the amount of salt in your diet. Do not add salt to your food and avoid eating processed foods, which are often high in salt. Be aware, though, that the reduction of salt will not help in all cases.

3. Increase your consumption of onions and garlic. In addition to its cholesterol-lowering and blood-thinning abilities, garlic also lowers blood pressure. Onions are also useful for this purpose.

Nutrients That Help

☐ **Calcium**, when present in high levels, is associated with low blood pressure.

☐ **Magnesium**, when present in low levels, is associated with high blood pressure.

☐ **Potassium**, when present in high levels, is associated with low blood pressure.

Beneficial Juices

☐ Kale, collard greens, and turnip greens—sources of calcium.

☐ Collard greens, parsley, and garlic—sources of magnesium.

☐ Celery, Swiss chard, carrot, and cantaloupe—sources of potassium.

☐ Onion and garlic—contain factors that lower blood pressure.

Suggested Juicing Recipes / Hypertension

Sweet Potassium Shake

¼ cantaloupe
1 banana

Juice cantaloupe. Place juice and banana in blender or food processor, and blend until smooth.

Sweet Calcium Shake

1 pint strawberries
6 oz. silken tofu

Juice strawberries. Place juice and tofu in blender or food processor, and blend until smooth. Garnish with strawberry.

Sweet Magnesium Smoothie

1 pint blackberries
1 ripe banana
2 oz. silken tofu
1 Tbsp. brewer's yeast

Juice berries. Place juice, banana, tofu, and yeast in blender or food processor, and blend until smooth. Garnish with blackberries. Drink 1 hour before bedtime.

Calcium-Rich Cocktail

3 kale leaves
Small handful parsley
4–5 carrots, greens removed
½ apple, seeded

Bunch up kale and parsley, and push through hopper with carrots and apple.

Potassium Broth

Handful parsley
Handful spinach
4–5 carrots, greens removed
2 stalks celery

Bunch up parsley and spinach leaves, and push through hopper with carrots and celery.

Harvest Soup

2–3 garlic cloves
1 kale leaf
1 large tomato
2 stalks celery
1 collard leaf, chopped
1 Tbsp. croutons

Roll garlic in kale leaf, and push through hopper with tomato and celery. Place juice in saucepan, add chopped collards, and gently heat. Garnish with croutons.

Garlic Express

Handful parsley
1 garlic clove
4–5 carrots, greens removed
2 stalks celery

Bunch up parsley and push through hopper with garlic, carrots, and celery.

Magnesium Drink

1 garlic clove
Small handful parsley
4–5 carrots, greens removed
2 stalks celery
Parsley sprig for garnish

Wrap garlic in parsley, and push through hopper with carrots and celery. Pour juice into glass, and garnish with sprig of parsley.

HYPOGLYCEMIA
(LOW BLOOD SUGAR)

Hypoglycemia is a disorder in which insulin is oversecreted by the pancreas, resulting in an abnormally low level of glucose (sugar) in the blood. This drop in the blood-sugar level deprives the brain of its main fuel—glucose—and the brain responds by producing a number of hormones, including adrenaline. It is the adrenaline that causes the symptoms of hypoglycemia: anxiety, shaking, sweating, and a racing heart. Many individuals also experience headaches, lack of concentration, tinnitus (unexplained sounds), and irritability. These symptoms are always relieved by eating a simple carbohydrate food. Treatment of hypoglycemia focuses on keeping blood-sugar levels even and supporting the pancreas.

Caution: Diabetics occasionally experience low blood sugar as a result of taking too much insulin. When this occurs, they should *not* follow the suggestions for hypoglycemia, but should contact their doctor immediately.

Dietary Recommendations

1. Follow the Sugar Metabolism Disorder Diet. (See page 288.) The diet for hypoglycemia is high in complex carbohydrates (55–60 percent of total calories) and low in protein (10–12 percent of total calories) and fat (30 percent of total calories). Eliminate white sugar and refined foods.

2. Eat foods rich in complex carbohydrates and soluble fiber, such as whole grain pasta, oat bran, beans, and lentils. These foods are digested slowly and raise blood glucose levels only slightly.

3. Eat smaller and more frequent meals.

4. Avoid coffee, tea, soft drinks containing caffeine, alcohol, and tobacco. These substances speed up the rate of digestion, releasing sugar into the blood stream at a faster rate.

5. Drink only very diluted fruit juices, no more than three glasses a week. Never eat anything that tastes sweet on an empty stomach.

6. Use cinnamon, cloves, bay leaves, and turmeric liberally. These spices have been shown to help regulate insulin activity.

7. If you experience a hypoglycemic reaction, do not eat foods high in sugar to relieve symptoms. Although this will initially cause your blood sugar to rise, afterward your sugar will plummet again as insulin is oversecreted in response to the sweets. This results in a ping-pong effect that leaves you feeling as though you are bouncing off the walls. Treat symptoms by eating a food that has a small amount of natural sugar and a lot of fiber to slow the sugar's release. (Beans are one such food.) This will relieve the symptoms as well as prevent recurrence.

Nutrients That Help

☐ **Chromium** helps regulate the effects of insulin in glucose metabolism. Research has not identified the form of chromium that the body needs for this purpose, so it is best to supplement this mineral by taking high-chromium brewer's yeast.

☐ **Insulin-promoting factor** improves glucose tolerance in animals that are chromium deficient. Foods high in this unidentified factor include tuna, peanut butter, clove, bay leaf, apple pie spice, cinnamon, and turmeric.

☐ **Manganese** is also involved in glucose metabolism.

Beneficial Juices

☐ Green pepper, apple, and spinach—sources of chromium.

☐ Turnip greens, beet greens, and carrot—sources of manganese.

Suggested Juicing Recipes / Hypoglycemia

Quick and Easy Soup

1 garlic clove
Handful spinach
2 stalks celery
½ cucumber
2 Tbsp. finely chopped turnip
   greens, beet greens, or
   spinach
1 Tbsp. brewer's yeast
Parsley sprig for garnish

Wrap garlic in spinach leaves, and push through hopper with celery and cucumber. Place juice in saucepan, add chopped vegetables, and gently warm. Sprinkle yeast on top and garnish with sprig of parsley. Serve hot.

Warm Apple Pie

1 tart apple, seeded
Water
Apple pie spice
Cinnamon stick for garnish

Juice apple. In small pan, bring 2 oz. juice and 4 oz. water to boil. Season with liberal amount of spice. Serve in teacup. Garnish with cinnamon stick.

Calcium-Rich Cocktail

3 kale leaves
Small handful parsley
4–5 carrots, greens removed
½ apple, seeded

Bunch up kale and parsley, and push through hopper with carrots and apple.

Pancreas Tonic

3 lettuce leaves
4–5 carrots, greens removed
Handful green beans
2 Brussels sprouts

Bunch up lettuce leaves and push through hopper with carrots, green beans, and Brussels sprouts.

Low-Sugar Pop

1 apple, seeded
¼ lime
Sparkling water

Juice apple and lime. Pour juice into tall, ice-filled glass. Fill glass to top with sparkling water.

Cucumber Cooler

1 tomato
1 cucumber
2 stalks celery
Parsley sprig for garnish

Juice tomato, pour juice into ice cube tray, and freeze. Juice cucumber and celery. Pour juice into tall glass, add tomato cubes, and garnish with sprig of parsley.

| **Popeye's Garden Tonic** |

Handful spinach
3 stalks celery
2 stalks asparagus
1 large tomato
1 cherry tomato for garnish

Bunch up spinach and push through hopper with celery. Juice asparagus and tomato. Mix juices in a tall glass and garnish with cherry tomato.

INDIGESTION

Indigestion, or dyspepsia, is a term that describes the symptoms of discomfort that accompany disorders of the digestive tract. Symptoms can include gas, abdominal pain, heartburn, a bloated feeling, and nausea. We list below some simple remedies, but remember that the cause of the symptoms must be found and treated if lasting relief is to be achieved. Indigestion can be caused by stress, eating too fast, not chewing food well, eating foods that are too high in fat, overeating, using medications (including over-the-counter medicines such as aspirin), drinking too much alcohol, using tobacco, and producing too much or too little stomach acid. Indigestion can also be a warning sign of a more serious problem. If it persists, be sure to see your physician.

General Recommendations

Stress reduction techniques may be beneficial. The elimination of tobacco and alcohol may be helpful, too; both of these substances irritate the stomach. See your physician for an evaluation of stomach acidity.

Dietary Modifications

1. Follow the Basic Diet. (See page 285.)

2. Eat small, frequent meals in a relaxed atmosphere, chewing your food thoroughly. Eat lightly during periods of stress.

3. Avoid coffee, which can cause symptoms of indigestion that may be mistaken for an ulcer. Both regular and decaffeinated coffee should be eliminated.

4. If low stomach acid (hypochlorhydria) is a problem, drink little or no liquid with meals, except fresh pineapple or papaya juice. Pineapple juice contains a protein-digesting enzyme called bromelain; papaya is a source of the enzyme papain. Both are considered digestive aids.

5. Drink a glass of water flavored with lemon juice one-half hour before meals. Fresh lemon juice is a traditional tonic for stimulating the appetite and increasing salivary and gastric secretions.

6. Heartburn, caused by stomach acid splashing into the esophagus, can often be controlled by eliminating alcohol, coffee, and chocolate, as well as carminatives (gas-relieving substances) such as peppermint oil, spearmint oil, and ginger. In some people, these substances relax the muscle at the top of the stomach, letting stomach acid leak.

7. If intestinal gas is causing pain, use carminatives such as peppermint oil to bring relief. In addition, gas caused by vegetables can be eliminated by using an enzyme product called Beano. This product, manufactured by the Lactaid Corporation, is available through your local pharmacy or health food store.

8. Stock up on ginger root. This root has been used as a carminative for thousands of years. Ginger can also be used as a remedy for morning sickness in pregnant women and to help prevent motion sickness. Recent reports indicate that ginger may protect the stomach lining from the damaging effects of nonsteroidal, anti-inflammatory drugs (NSAID) such as aspirin and Naprosyn (naproxen).

9. Drink cabbage juice. The ulcer-healing factor in fresh cabbage juice works for gastritis as well. (See ULCERS in Part Two for more information.)

10. Eat bananas. Animal studies have shown that bananas can protect the stomach from stomach acids.

11. See also COLITIS and DIARRHEA in Part Two.

Nutrients That Help

☐ **Bromelain** is a protein-digesting enzyme.

☐ **Papain** is a protein-digesting enzyme.

Beneficial Juices

☐ Cabbage and celery—sources of the ulcer-healing factor.

☐ Ginger—contains a carminative that also protects the stomach.

☐ Pineapple—only source of the enzyme bromelain.

☐ Papaya—fresh juice from the unripe fruit contains the enzyme papain.

☐ Kiwi—fresh juice contains a digestive enzyme.

☐ Lemon—a traditional appetite stimulant.

Suggested Juicing Recipes / Indigestion

Lemon Spritzer

1 small lemon	Push lemon through hopper.
Sparkling water	Pour juice into ice-filled glass.
	Fill glass to top with
	sparkling water.

Heartburn Quencher

¼ head cabbage	Juice vegetables. Drink three
1 stalk celery	times a day.
2 carrots, greens removed	

Tropical Squeeze

1 firm papaya, peeled	Juice papaya. Push ginger
¼-inch slice ginger root	through hopper with pear.
1 pear	

Kiwi Crush

1 firm kiwi, peeled
1 green apple, seeded
1 small bunch grapes
Kiwi slice for garnish

Push kiwi through hopper with apple and grapes. Pour juice into tall, ice-filled glass. Garnish with kiwi slice.

Monkey Shake

½ orange, peeled (leave white pithy part)
½ papaya, peeled
1 banana
Orange twist for garnish

Push orange through hopper with papaya. Place juice and banana in blender or food processor, and blend until smooth. Garnish with orange twist.

Digestive Aid

¼ pineapple, with skin

Juice pineapple. Drink with meals as your only fluid.

Ginger Fizz

¼-inch slice ginger root
1 apple, seeded
Sparkling water

Push ginger through hopper with apple. Pour juice into ice-filled glass. Fill glass to top with sparkling water.

Garden Tonic

¼ head cabbage
2 stalks celery
1 stalk broccoli
Parsley sprig for garnish

Juice vegetables and garnish with sprig of parsley.

INFECTIONS

Infection is the invasion of the body by foreign organisms. Your body has an army designed to identify and destroy harmful invaders. This army is called the immune system. Like all armies, your immune system marches on its stomach. Keep your immune soldiers well provisioned using the ideas listed below. Remember that over-the-counter "flu" remedies work by masking flu symptoms. The natural remedies outlined here work by making your immune soldiers stronger so they can protect your cells from infection more effectively.

General Recommendations

When sick, go to bed if at all possible. Sleep gives your immune system a chance to renew itself. If a cough, sore throat, or fever does not respond to the treatment here, call your physician. Antibiotics may be necessary for the treatment of bacterial infections. Since antibiotics can destroy the colon's beneficial bacteria, be sure to include a source of acidophilus bacteria in your diet. Aspirin has been associated with a rare disorder called Reye's Syndrome, which usually affects people under eighteen years of age. Never give aspirin to a child or teen who has any kind of infection.

Dietary Modifications

1. Follow the Immune Support Diet. (See page 293.)

2. Limit the amount of sweet-tasting foods you eat or drink, including fruit juice. That's right, even orange juice is a no-no when you have an infection. Sugar decreases the ability of your white blood cells to destroy bacteria and viruses.

3. Drink large amounts of fluids, like diluted vegetable juices and broths, or just plain water. For those over seventeen years of age, a Juice Fast may be beneficial during the first one or two days. (See page 301.)

4. *Add garlic to your diet.* The allicin component of garlic is an effective antibiotic.

5. *Increase your consumption of cabbage, which stimulates the body to produce more antibodies to combat infections.* In the test tube, cabbage actually kills viruses and bacteria.

6. *Anthocyanins are anutrients with antiviral and antibacterial action.* These compounds are found in high concentrations in blueberries and black currants.

7. *Tannins are another nutrient that kills viruses in the test tube.* Grape tannins are particularly effective at killing the herpes simplex virus.

8. *Increase your consumption of apples and apple juice, which have been linked to a lower incidence of colds in college students.* Apple juice has been shown to have anti-viral properties.

9. *See also* CANDIDIASIS, CHRONIC FATIGUE SYNDROME, COMMON COLD, HERPES SIMPLEX I AND II, and SORE THROAT in Part Two.

Nutrients That Help

☐ **Potassium** is lost during bouts of fever, vomiting, and diarrhea.

☐ **Sodium** is lost during bouts of fever, vomiting, and diarrhea.

☐ **Vitamin C** stimulates the immune system in a number of different ways, as well as being antiviral and antibacterial.

☐ **Bioflavonoids** enhance the effects of vitamin C, as well as being antiviral.

☐ **Beta-carotene** is a potent immune strengthener that also has antiviral properties.

☐ **Zinc** is very important for the proper functioning of the immune system's natural killer cells.

Beneficial Juices

☐ Blueberry and black currant—contain antibacterial agents that are also antidiarrheal.

☐ Grape, apple, and cabbage—contain antiviral and antibacterial compounds.

☐ Garlic—the most potent natural antibiotic.

☐ Pineapple—fresh juice contains the enzyme bromelain, which is an effective anti-inflammatory agent for sore throats.

☐ Celery, carrot, and Swiss chard—contain high amounts of potassium and sodium.

☐ Kale, red pepper, and collard greens—low-sugar sources of vitamin C.

☐ Tomato, cabbage, and sweet pepper—low-sugar sources of bioflavonoids.

☐ Carrot, kale, and spinach—low-sugar sources of beta-carotene.

☐ Ginger, parsley, and carrot—sources of zinc.

Suggested Juicing Recipes / Infections

Immune Builder

Handful parsley
1 garlic clove
5 carrots, greens removed
3 stalks celery

Bunch up parsley, and push through hopper with garlic, carrots, and celery.

Potassium Broth

Handful parsley
Handful spinach
4–5 carrots, greens removed
2 stalks celery

Bunch up parsley and spinach leaves, and push through hopper with carrots and celery.

Christmas Cocktail

2 apples, seeded
1 large bunch grapes
1 lemon wedge

*Push apples, grapes, and
lemon through hopper.*

Bluemint Fizz

Handful mint
1 pint blueberries
Sparkling water
Mint sprig for garnish

*Bunch up mint and push
through hopper with berries.
Pour juice into tall, ice-filled
glass. Fill glass to top with
sparkling water. Garnish with
sprig of mint.*

Low-Sugar Pop

1 apple, seeded
¼ lime
Sparkling water

*Juice apple and lime. Pour
juice into tall, ice-filled glass.
Fill glass to top with
sparkling water.*

Sweet and Sour Cherry Cream

1 cup cherries, pitted
4 oz. nonfat yogurt

*Juice cherries. Place juice and
yogurt in blender or food
processor, and blend until
smooth.*

Pineapple Protein Shake

3 pineapple rings, with skin
4 oz. soymilk
1 ripe banana
2–3 Tbsp. protein powder
Pineapple spear for garnish

*Juice pineapple. Place juice,
soymilk, banana, and protein
powder into blender or food
processor, and blend until
smooth. Pour juice into tall
glass and garnish with
pineapple spear.*

Harvest Soup

2–3 garlic cloves
1 kale leaf
1 large tomato
2 stalks celery
1 collard leaf, chopped
1 Tbsp. croutons

Roll garlic in kale leaf, and push through hopper with tomato and celery. Place juice in saucepan, add chopped collards, and gently heat. Garnish with croutons.

INFLAMMATION

Inflammation is the response of living tissue to injury. The injury can be caused by bacteria or virus, surgery, or an accident. We are all familiar with the symptoms of inflammation—redness, pain, swelling, and heat. These symptoms are not caused by the injury itself, but are the result of the mobilization of our body's protective system, the immune army, to bring aid to the injured area. Inflammation can be helpful (as when you have a bacterial infection) or harmful (as in arthritis). The natural remedies below can help by reducing inflammation, and thereby lessening some of the painful effects, without decreasing the helpful aspects of the response.

General Recommendations

For inflammation caused by injury, try **RIP**: **R**est, **I**ce, and **P**rotection. Rest the injured area, apply ice wrapped in a towel for thirty minutes, and then protect the injured area until you can see a doctor. Ice can be applied for thirty minutes on, fifteen minutes off, for up to eight hours if swelling continues. After the first twenty-four hours, heat may be applied.

For inflammation caused by disease—such as an autoimmune disease like arthritis—an elimination diet may identify food allergies. Inflammation, in this instance, is caused by a response of the immune system to an imagined invader. Overstimulation of the immune system by allergies is felt by some researchers to make symptoms worse.

Dietary Modifications

1. *Follow the Immune Support Diet.* (See page 293.)

2. *If you suspect that allergies may be aggravating your condition, try the Elimination Diet.* (See page 296.)

3. *Eat a diet high in fatty cold-water fish such as mackerel, herring, and salmon.* In one study, the omega-3 fatty acids found in these fish were shown to reduce the symptoms of inflammatory skin disorders.

4. *Add ginger to your diet.* Ginger may protect the stomach from ulcers caused by nonsteroidal anti-inflammatory drugs (NSAID). Ginger also has anti-inflammatory properties.

5. *Add pineapple to your diet.* Bromelain, an enzyme found only in fresh pineapple, has anti-inflammatory properties. Whenever there is inflammation, think pineapple.

6. *For swollen sinuses, avoid dairy products, except plain yogurt, and drink hot liquids to reduce the congestion and sinus pressure.*

7. *See also* ARTHRITIS, CARPAL TUNNEL SYNDROME, and SORE THROAT in Part Two.

Nutrients That Help

☐ **Bioflavonoids** inhibit the release of histamine, a substance that's released in response to infections and allergic reactions.

☐ **Vitamin C** stabilizes cell membranes and contains an antihistamine.

☐ **Vitamin E** has anti-inflammatory actions.

☐ **Zinc** is involved in many anti-inflammatory processes.

☐ **Omega-3 fatty acids**, found in cold-water fatty fish, reduce inflammation by lessening prostaglandin synthesis.

☐ **Omega-6 fatty acids**, found in evening primrose oil, have been shown to reduce acute inflammatory reactions.

Beneficial Juices

☐ Ginger—an anti-inflammatory agent itself, this root also protects the stomach from the effects of nonsteroidal anti-inflammatory drugs (NSAID).

☐ Pineapple—fresh juice contains the anti-inflammatory enzyme bromelain.

☐ Red pepper, parsley, and orange—sources of vitamin C and bioflavonoids.

☐ Spinach, asparagus, and kiwi—sources of vitamin E.

☐ Parsley, garlic, and carrot—sources of zinc.

Suggested Juicing Recipes / Inflammation

Hawaiian Fizz

3 pineapple rings, with skin	*Juice pineapple. Push ginger*
1/4-inch slice ginger root	*through hopper with pear.*
1/2 pear	*Pour juice into a tall glass*
Sparkling water	*and fill with sparkling water.*
Pineapple spear for garnish	*Garnish with pineapple spear.*

Ginger Hopper

1/4-inch slice ginger root	*Push ginger through hopper*
4–5 carrots, greens removed	*with carrots and apple.*
1/2 apple, seeded	

Popeye's Garden Tonic

Handful spinach	*Bunch up spinach and push*
3 stalks celery	*through hopper with celery.*
2 stalks asparagus	*Juice asparagus and tomato.*
1 large tomato	*Mix juices in a tall glass and*
1 cherry tomato for garnish	*garnish with cherry tomato.*

Tossed Salad

1 kale leaf
1 turnip leaf
Handful spinach
2 tomatoes
1 cherry tomato for garnish

Bunch up the leaves and spinach, and push through hopper with tomatoes. Garnish with cherry tomato.

Orange Spice Tea

½-inch ginger root
1 orange, peeled (leave white pithy part)
Water
Cinnamon stick for garnish

Push ginger and orange through hopper. Pour 2 oz. of juice into teacup and fill with boiling water. Garnish with cinnamon stick.

Garlic Express

Handful parsley
1 garlic clove
4–5 carrots, greens removed
2 stalks celery

Bunch up parsley and push through hopper with garlic, carrots, and celery.

INSOMNIA

Insomnia is defined as difficulty in falling asleep or frequent or early awakening. This extremely frustrating problem affects everybody at some time. Psychological problems are the cause of 50 percent of all sleep difficulties. Drugs such as thyroid preparations, beta blockers, marijuana, caffeine, and alcohol can also prevent or disrupt sleep.

General Recommendations

Whatever works safely, use. Regular exercise helps to promote deep sleep, and it is also a means of reducing daily stress.

Dealing with psychological problems through counseling is also a good idea. If you are taking any medications, ask your doctor or pharmacist if they might be causing your insomnia.

Dietary Modifications

1. Follow the Basic Diet. (See page 285.)

2. Remove caffeine-containing beverages such as coffee, tea, and colas from your diet. Replace them with some of the nerve-soothing juices listed below.

3. Do not drink alcohol. Some people have a drink or two at bedtime to relax. This may help you fall asleep, but it may also wake you up after a few hours because alcohol disrupts sleep patterns.

4. Consider nighttime hypoglycemia as a possible cause of your problem. See HYPOGLYCEMIA in Part Two.

5. Drink a high-glucose or high-sucrose fruit juice before going to bed. This may help to increase levels of serotonin, a sleep-inducing brain chemical. Try this only if you are sure hypoglycemia is not a problem.

Nutrients That Help

☐ **Niacin, vitamin B6, and magnesium** are cofactors in the conversion of the amino acid tryptophan into the sleep-inducing chemical serotonin.

☐ **Calcium** aids in muscle relaxation.

☐ **Folate** may help alleviate restless leg syndrome, a problem that can contribute to insomnia.

Beneficial Juices

☐ Broccoli, tomato, and carrot—sources of niacin.

☐ Spinach, carrot, and pea—good sources of vitamin B6.

☐ Parsley, collard greens, and blackberry—sources of magnesium.

☐ Kale, collard greens, and broccoli—good sources of calcium.

☐ Asparagus, spinach, and kale—good sources of folate.

☐ Lettuce and celery—traditional remedies for insomnia.

☐ Grape and pineapple—high in glucose and sucrose.

Suggested Juicing Recipes / Insomnia

Traditional Sleep Potion

3–4 lettuce leaves 1 stalk celery	*Bunch up lettuce and push through hopper with celery. Drink 30 minutes before bedtime.*

Calcium-Rich Cocktail

3 kale leaves Small handful parsley 4–5 carrots, greens removed ½ apple, seeded	*Bunch up kale and parsley, and push through hopper with carrots and apple.*

Popeye's Garden Tonic

Handful spinach 3 stalks celery 2 stalks asparagus 1 large tomato 1 cherry tomato for garnish	*Bunch up spinach and push through hopper with celery. Juice asparagus and tomato. Mix juices in a tall glass and garnish with cherry tomato.*

Sweet Magnesium Smoothie

1 pint blackberries 1 ripe banana 2 oz. silken tofu 1 Tbsp. brewer's yeast	*Juice berries. Place juice, banana, tofu, and yeast in blender or food processor, and blend until smooth. Garnish with blackberries. Drink 1 hour before bedtime.*

Traditional Nerve Soother

1 stalk celery
3–4 carrots, greens removed

Juice celery and carrots.
Drink 1 hour before bedtime.

Bromelain Special

¼ pineapple, with skin

Push pineapple through
hopper.

Garden Salad Special

3 broccoli flowerets
1 garlic clove
4–5 carrots or 2 tomatoes
2 stalks celery
½ green pepper

Push broccoli and garlic
through hopper with carrots
or tomatoes. Follow with
celery and green pepper.

IRRITABLE BOWEL SYNDROME

See COLITIS.

LOW BLOOD SUGAR

See HYPOGLYCEMIA.

LYME DISEASE

The name of this disease comes from the town of Lyme, Connecticut, the site of its first discovery. It is found mostly in areas where white-tail deer live. A small tick carried by the deer transmits Lyme disease, and household pets can carry the tick into the home, where it is transmitted to the human residents. Walking in forested areas can also expose a person to the tick. In the eastern United States, the primary host is the white-footed field mouse. In the western states, the tick is carried by lizards and jack rabbits. If tick bites go undetected, the disease can develop. One of the first signs is a rash that appears a few days after the bite, followed by a red papule on the skin. Other possible symptoms include fever, chills, nausea, and vomiting. It is imperative to see a doctor as soon as these symptoms appear. Your doctor will be able to perform a blood test to identify the condition. If left untreated, Lyme disease can cause arthritis and damage the cardiovascular and central nervous systems. Signs of this include fatigue, flu-like symptoms, stiff neck, headache, vomiting, and nausea.

General Recommendations

There is now antibiotic therapy for Lyme disease. In addition, you can support your immune system nutritionally. To relieve joint pain, try heat in the form of hot baths or a whirlpool. Finally, try to avoid stressful situations as much as possible because of their devastating effects on the immune system.

Dietary Modifications

1. *Follow the Immune Support Diet.* (See page 293.)

2. *Avoid all simple sugars, including glucose, fructose, sucrose, honey, maple syrup, fruit juice concentrate, corn syrup, dextrose, and all other sweeteners.* Also avoid drinking orange juice because of its high sugar content. Sweeteners depress the immune system. Avoid artificial sweeteners, too. And have a long talk with your "sweet tooth" about how much you want to get well! If you still crave sweets, try to eliminate your cravings through diet. (*See* CRAVINGS in Part Two.)

3. *Generously include garlic and ginger root in your diet.* These foods act as natural antibiotics and are potent immune stimulators.

Nutrients That Help

☐ **Beta-carotene**, which is converted by your body to vitamin A, stimulates numerous immune processes. Beta-carotene is an excellent antioxidant.

☐ **Vitamin B6** deficiency results in depressed immunity.

☐ **Vitamin C**, which is rapidly depleted from white blood cells (your first line of defense) during infections, has antiviral and antibacterial properties.

☐ **Vitamin E** is an important antioxidant.

☐ **Zinc** is a critical nutrient of immunity.

☐ **Selenium** is an important antioxidant.

☐ **Chlorophyll**, a blood purifier, can be beneficial.

Beneficial Juices

☐ Carrot, kale, parsley, and spinach—sources of beta-carotene.

☐ Kale, spinach, and sweet pepper—sources of vitamin B6.

☐ Kale, parsley, green pepper, and broccoli—sources of vitamin C.

☐ Spinach, asparagus, and carrot—sources of vitamin E.

☐ Ginger root, parsley, potassium, garlic, and carrot—sources of zinc.

☐ Turnip, garlic, radish, and grape—sources of selenium.

☐ Green vegetables—sources of chlorophyll.

Suggested Juicing Recipes / Lyme Disease

Ginger Hopper

¼-inch slice ginger root
4–5 carrots, greens removed
½ apple, seeded

Push ginger through hopper with carrots and apple.

Immune Builder

Handful parsley
1 garlic clove
5 carrots, greens removed
3 stalks celery

*Bunch up parsley, and push
through hopper with garlic,
carrots, and celery.*

Garden Salad Special

3 broccoli flowerets
1 garlic clove
4–5 carrots or 2 tomatoes
2 stalks celery
½ green pepper

*Push broccoli and garlic
through hopper with carrots
or tomatoes. Follow with
celery and green pepper.*

Tomato Salad Express

Handful spinach
Handful parsley
2 tomatoes
½ green pepper
Dash Tabasco sauce

*Bunch up spinach and
parsley, and push through
hopper with tomatoes and
green pepper. Add Tabasco
sauce.*

Christmas Cocktail

2 apples, seeded
1 large bunch grapes
1 lemon wedge

*Push apples, grapes, and
lemon through hopper.*

Mineral Tonic

Handful parsley
2 turnip leaves
1 kale leaf
4–5 carrots, greens removed

*Roll up parsley in turnip and
kale leaves, and push
through hopper with carrots.*

MEMORY LOSS

At one time or another, each of us has experienced an unexplained loss of mental ability. Unfortunately, a decrease in
memory or thinking ability is often passed off as being "normal" for the older person. Nonsense, we say! The brain is very
sensitive to the health status of the body. When your body is
run down, your brain is sure to follow. A nutrient-deficient
diet, hormone imbalance, glandular disorder, or heavy-metal
toxicity from lead or mercury can all cause memory problems.
If you occasionally spend an hour searching the house for the
sunglasses on your head, try some of the ideas below. They
may help to clear the fog.

General Recommendations

Stress, food allergies, and hypoglycemia can all cause "foggy"
thinking. Sometimes, vitamin deficiency is to blame. Vitamin
B_{12} is often poorly absorbed in the later years, and supplementation by injection may dramatically clear the head. If you
suspect a physical disorder such as hormone imbalance or
heavy-metal toxicity, see your physician.

Dietary Modifications

1. *Follow the Basic Diet.* (See page 285.) This diet will help
to rebuild your body and brain.

**2. *If you need to remember what you are reading, snack
on a food that is high in fat.*** Fat stimulates the release of
the neurotransmitter cholecystokinin, which may help to "fix"
the information in your memory. Seeds and nut butters are
the best choices here because of their "healthful" oil content.

3. *See also* ALLERGIES, HYPOGLYCEMIA, and STRESS in Part Two.

Nutrients That Help

☐ **Thiamin** is often called the nerve vitamin. Even a mild deficit of this nutrient has been linked with some impairment of brain activity. Yeast, wheat germ, and sunflower seeds are all high in thiamin.

☐ **Riboflavin** has been linked with mental ability. People with adequate amounts of this B vitamin performed better on memory tests than did people with inadequate levels of this nutrient.

☐ **Carotene** has been linked with improved memory. People with adequate amounts of this orange pigment did better on thinking or cognitive tests than those who were only slightly deficient.

☐ **Vitamin B**$_{12}$ deficiency has been linked with memory problems. Low levels of this vitamin were associated with low scores on a test. Animal proteins are the best source of this vitamin.

☐ **Folate** deficiency has been linked with memory problems. Low levels of this nutrient were associated with low scores on a test.

☐ **Iron** has been linked with excellent mental ability. Older adults with high iron status have shown the same brain wave activity as young adults.

☐ **Vitamin C** increases absorption of iron.

Beneficial Juices

☐ Collard greens, kale, and parsley—sources of riboflavin.

☐ Carrot, kale, and cantaloupe—excellent sources of carotene.

☐ Asparagus, spinach, and kale—sources of folate.

☐ Kale and parsley—good sources of iron.

☐ Red pepper, kale, and parsley—good sources of vitamin C.

Suggested Juicing Recipes / Memory Loss

Peach Nectar

2 firm peaches, pitted   *Juice peaches and lime. Place*
1/2 lime   *juice, banana, and yeast in*
1 ripe banana   *blender or food processor,*
1 Tbsp. brewer's yeast   *and blend until smooth.*

Cantaloupe Shake

½ cantaloupe, with skin   *Cut cantaloupe in strips, and*
                                push through hopper.

Green Surprise

1 large kale leaf   *Bunch up kale leaf and push*
2–3 green apples, seeded   *through hopper with apples.*
Lime twist for garnish   *Garnish with lime twist. The*
                                surprise is that you won't
                                taste the kale!

Brain Booster

1 large tart apple, seeded   *Juice apple. Place juice and*
1 cup cashew nuts   *nuts in blender or food*
                                processor, and blend until
                                smooth. Chill until mixture
                                thickens. Serve on whole
                                wheat crackers.

Harvest Soup

2–3 garlic cloves   *Roll garlic in kale leaf, and*
1 kale leaf   *push through hopper with*
1 large tomato   *tomato and celery. Place juice*
2 stalks celery   *in saucepan, add chopped*
1 collard leaf, chopped   *collards, and gently heat.*
1 Tbsp. croutons   *Garnish with croutons.*

Mineral Tonic

Handful parsley
2 turnip leaves
1 kale leaf
4–5 carrots, greens removed

*Roll up parsley in turnip and
kale leaves, and push
through hopper with carrots.*

Popeye's Garden Tonic

Handful spinach
3 stalks celery
2 stalks asparagus
1 large tomato
1 cherry tomato for garnish

*Bunch up spinach and push
through hopper with celery.
Juice asparagus and tomato.
Mix juices in a tall glass and
garnish with cherry tomato.*

MENOPAUSAL SYMPTOMS

Menopause is the point at which women stop ovulating. Contrary to popular opinion, the female body does not stop producing hormones after menopause. For instance, the adrenal glands continue to produce androgens, the hormones responsible for the sex drive. However, levels of the estrogen estradiol drop to one-tenth their previous levels. It is the decrease of this type of estrogen that is thought to be responsible for the symptoms of menopause, with hot flashes, night sweats, and vaginal dryness being the most common problems. Diet can help minimize the symptoms of menopause. So, plug in your juicer and make your "change of life" a change for the better.

General Recommendations

Your risk of developing heart disease and osteoporosis increases after menopause. For this reason, you may want to learn more about these disorders and take steps to reduce the risks. (*See* ATHEROSCLEROSIS and OSTEOPOROSIS in Part Two.) A water-soluble lubricant such as K-Y jelly will help to relieve vaginal dryness. Some women find that hot flashes respond well to acupuncture. Most important, get outside and walk. Exercise will help to prevent osteoporosis and heart disease.

Dietary Modifications

1. Follow the Basic Diet. (See page 285.)

2. Increase your consumption of soy foods, such as soymilk, tofu, and tempeh. Soy foods contain plant estrogens that supplement the estrogens made by the ovaries.

3. Reduce the amount of fat in your diet. This will help to decrease your risk of heart disease.

Nutrients That Help

☐ **Bioflavonoids** help to reduce symptoms.

☐ **Vitamin E** may reduce hot flashes. Sunflower seeds, almonds, and wheat germ are excellent sources of this vitamin.

☐ **Magnesium** is involved in bone formation and is necessary to prevent osteoporosis.

☐ **Calcium** is involved in bone formation and is necessary to prevent osteoporosis.

Beneficial Juices

☐ Orange, tomato, cabbage, and grapefruit—sources of bioflavonoids.

☐ Spinach, asparagus, and kiwi—sources of vitamin E.

☐ Collard greens, parsley, and blackberry—sources of magnesium.

☐ Kale, collard greens, and parsley—excellent sources of calcium.

Suggested Juicing Recipes / Menopausal Symptoms

Sweet Calcium Shake

---

1 pint strawberries
6 oz. silken tofu

Juice strawberries. Place juice and tofu in blender or food processor, and blend until smooth. Garnish with strawberry.

Super-Eight Stress Reliever

---

1 kale leaf
1 collard leaf
Small handful parsley
1 stalk celery
1 carrot, greens removed
½ red pepper
1 tomato
1 broccoli floweret
Celery stalk for garnish

Bunch up leaves and parsley, and push through hopper with celery and carrot. Follow with red pepper, tomato, and broccoli. Garnish with celery stalk.

Sweet Magnesium Smoothie

---

1 pint blackberries
1 ripe banana
2 oz. silken tofu
1 Tbsp. brewer's yeast

Juice berries. Place juice, banana, tofu, and yeast in blender or food processor, and blend until smooth. Garnish with blackberries. Drink 1 hour before bedtime.

Popeye's Garden Tonic

Handful spinach
3 stalks celery
2 stalks asparagus
1 large tomato
1 cherry tomato for garnish

Bunch up spinach and push through hopper with celery. Juice asparagus and tomato. Mix juices in a tall glass and garnish with cherry tomato.

Calcium-Rich Cocktail

3 kale leaves
Small handful parsley
4–5 carrots, greens removed
½ apple, seeded

*Bunch up kale and parsley,
and push through hopper
with carrots and apple.*

Spiced Orange Foam

¼-inch slice ginger root
2 large oranges, peeled (leave
    white pithy part)
½ apple, seeded
Orange twist for garnish

*Push ginger through hopper
with orange and apple. Serve
with twist of orange.*

Garden Tonic

¼ head cabbage
2 stalks celery
1 stalk broccoli
Parsley sprig for garnish

*Juice vegetables and garnish
with sprig of parsley.*

Orange Spice Tea

½-inch ginger root
1 orange, peeled (leave white
    pithy part)
Water
Cinnamon stick for garnish

*Push ginger and orange
through hopper. Pour 2 oz. of
juice into teacup and fill with
boiling water. Garnish with
cinnamon stick.*

MENSTRUAL PROBLEMS

Long, heavy periods are a problem for many women, causing a loss of many important minerals. Fortunately, this disorder responds well to nutritional intervention. The dietary suggestions that follow can help to lessen menstrual bleeding and to alleviate menstrual pain.

General Recommendations

Have your physician check your thyroid function. Even a mildly underactive thyroid can cause menstrual difficulties.

Dietary Modifications

1. *Follow the Basic Diet.* (See page 285.)

2. *Eat a diet that's low in animal fats.* Animal fats contain a fatty acid that increases the release of series 2 prostaglandins, which may be the cause of heavy cramping and bleeding.

Nutrients That Help

☐ **Iron** deficiency can be caused by menstruation and, in addition, can *be* the cause of excessive menstrual bleeding and cramping.

☐ **Vitamin C and bioflavonoids** strengthen capillaries, reduce bleeding, and increase the absorption of iron.

☐ **Vitamin K** in a **chlorophyll** extract reduced bleeding in several studies.

☐ **Magnesium** has relieved uterine muscle spasms.

☐ **Bromelain** has anti-inflammatory properties and is a smooth-muscle relaxant.

Beneficial Juices

☐ Kale and parsley—sources of both iron and vitamin C.

☐ Cherry, grape, lemon, and tomato—sources of bioflavonoids.

☐ Turnip greens, broccoli, and cabbage—sources of vitamin K and chlorophyll.

☐ Collard greens, parsley, and garlic—sources of magnesium.

☐ Pineapple—a source of bromelain.

Suggested Juicing Recipes / Menstrual Problems

Mineral Tonic

Handful parsley
2 turnip leaves
1 kale leaf
4–5 carrots, greens removed

Roll up parsley in turnip and kale leaves, and push through hopper with carrots.

Sweet Magnesium Smoothie

1 pint blackberries
1 ripe banana
2 oz. silken tofu
1 Tbsp. brewer's yeast

Juice berries. Place juice, banana, tofu, and yeast in blender or food processor, and blend until smooth. Garnish with blackberries. Drink 1 hour before bedtime.

Maureen's Spicy Tonic

¼ pineapple, with skin
½ apple, seeded
¼-inch slice ginger root

Push pineapple through hopper with apple and ginger.

Sweet and Sour Red Pop

½ lemon
1 pint cherries, pitted
Sparkling water

Juice lemon. Pour juice into ice cube tray, add water, and freeze. Juice cherries. Pour juice into tall glass, add lemon-juice cubes, and fill to top with sparkling water.

Garden Tonic

¼ head cabbage
2 stalks celery
1 stalk broccoli
Parsley sprig for garnish

Juice vegetables and garnish with sprig of parsley.

K-Cooler

1 turnip green   *Juice vegetables and apple.*
1 stalk broccoli   *Pour juice into ice-filled glass,*
1 red apple, seeded   *and garnish with parsley.*
Parsley sprig for garnish

Magnesium Drink

1 garlic clove   *Wrap garlic in parsley, and*
Small handful parsley   *push through hopper with*
4–5 carrots, greens removed   *carrots and celery. Pour juice*
2 stalks celery   *into glass, and garnish with*
Parsley sprig for garnish   *sprig of parsley.*

MIGRAINE HEADACHE

The connection between diet and headache has been suspected since the time of Hippocrates. Migraine headaches cause severe throbbing pain on one or both sides of the head, and may be accompanied by nausea and vomiting. Other common symptoms include sensitivity to light, tingling, dizziness, ringing in the ears, chills, and sweating. This kind of headache often causes its sufferers to take to bed in a darkened room, and can last anywhere from two hours to three days. Migraines appear to be caused by the contraction and sudden dilation of the blood vessels inside the brain. In many individuals, this process can be triggered by foods. Treatment consists of identifying the offending substances that trigger the headache and eliminating them from the diet. This involves some detective work, but the results are well worth the effort.

General Recommendations

Biofeedback classes can help some people reduce the severity and length of their migraines. Feverfew, an herb, is also effective for some individuals.

Dietary Modifications

1. *Follow the Basic Diet.* (See page 285.)

2. *Investigate the possibility of a food allergy or food intolerance.* Research indicates that food allergies may be a major cause of migraine headaches. Use the Elimination Diet (see page 296) to identify foods that may be causing allergic reactions.

3. *Avoid foods containing tyramine.* This naturally occurring substance can cause vasodilation (widening of the blood vessels) in some individuals. It has been estimated that up to 10 percent of migraine sufferers are sensitive to tyramine. Tyramine-containing foods include all alcoholic beverages, and red wine in particular; homemade yeast breads; sour cream; aged cheese; red plums; figs; aged game; liver, including chicken liver; canned meats; salami; sausage; salted dried fish; pickled herring; Italian broad beans; green bean pods; eggplant; soy sauce; and yeast concentrates, found in soup cubes, commercial gravies, and meat extracts.

4. *Avoid other foods that commonly trigger migraines.* These foods include cow's milk; goat's milk; wheat; chocolate; eggs; oranges; benzoic acid; tomatoes; tartrazine (a food coloring); rye; rice; fish; oats; cane sugar; yeast; grapes; onion; soy; pork; peanuts; walnuts; beef; tea; coffee; nuts; and corn.

5. *Eliminate sources of monosodium glutamate (MSG) from your diet.* This food additive causes headaches in susceptible individuals. Used as a flavor enhancer, it is frequently found in frozen and packaged processed foods and Chinese restaurant dishes.

6. *Discontinue the use of aspartame (NutraSweet).* This sugar substitute causes severe headaches in some people.

7. *Increase your consumption of foods that reduce platelet stickiness, such as cold-water fatty fish like mackerel, salmon, sardines, and anchovies.* Platelets are the blood cells that are responsible for blood clotting. Foods that inhibit blood clotting have been shown to reduce migraines.

Nutrients That Help

☐ **Magnesium** is a smooth-muscle relaxant.

☐ **Omega-3 fatty acids** inhibit blood clotting, reducing the incidence and severity of migraines. Your best source of this nutrient is cold-water fatty fish.

Beneficial Juices

☐ Collard greens, garlic, and parsley—sources of magnesium.

☐ Ginger root, cantaloupe, and garlic—reduce platelet stickiness.

Suggested Juicing Recipes / Migraine Headache

Spicy Cantaloupe Shake

¼-inch slice ginger root
½ cantaloupe, with skin

Push ginger through hopper with cantaloupe.

Magnesium Drink

1 garlic clove
Small handful parsley
4–5 carrots, greens removed
2 stalks celery
Parsley sprig for garnish

Wrap garlic in parsley, and push through hopper with carrots and celery. Pour juice into glass, and garnish with sprig of parsley.

Instant Soup

2–3 garlic cloves
1 bunch spinach
½ cucumber
1 stalk celery
2 Tbsp. finely chopped
    spinach and celery
Parsley sprig for garnish

Wrap garlic cloves in spinach, and push through hopper with cucumber and celery. Place juice in pan, add chopped vegetables, and gently heat. Garnish with sprig of parsley. Serve hot.

Ginger Hopper

¼-inch slice ginger root
4–5 carrots, greens removed
½ apple, seeded

Push ginger through hopper with carrots and apple.

Ginger Fizz

¼-inch slice ginger root
1 apple, seeded
Sparkling water

Push ginger through hopper with apple. Pour juice into ice-filled glass. Fill glass to top with sparkling water.

Ginger Tea

2-inch slice ginger root
¼ lemon
1 pint water
1 stick cinnamon, broken
4–5 cloves
Dash nutmeg or cardamom

Juice ginger and lemon. Place juice in saucepan, and add water, cinnamon, and cloves. Gently simmer. Add nutmeg or cardamom.

Sweet Magnesium Smoothie

1 pint blackberries
1 ripe banana
2 oz. silken tofu
1 Tbsp. brewer's yeast

Juice berries. Place juice, banana, tofu, and yeast in blender or food processor, and blend until smooth. Garnish with blackberries. Drink 1 hour before bedtime.

Waldorf Salad

1 green apple, seeded
1 stalk celery

Push apple and celery through hopper.

MOTION SICKNESS

Does the thought of a car trip turn you green? Can you feel the ocean waves crashing in your stomach when you venture out in a boat? If you can, you are one of the many people who experience symptoms that range from severe headache to dizziness, nausea, and vomiting while flying, sailing, or traveling in automobiles, buses, or trains. Skip the over-the-counter drugs; they can leave you sleepy. Try these natural "fixes"; they are as gentle as they are effective. If you suddenly find yourself prone to motion sickness when you have never had trouble before, see your doctor. It may be an indication of an inner ear problem.

General Recommendations

Avoid cigarette smoke, yours and other people's. Avoid food odors and overheated, stuffy rooms. If at sea, lie down and close your eyes at the first sign of motion sickness.

Dietary Modifications

1. Eat lightly when traveling. Avoid high-fat and high-sugar foods.

2. Eliminate alcohol from your diet. It can irritate an already stressed stomach.

3. Pack one of the ginger drinks (see recipes at the end of this section) in a thermos and bring it along with you.

4. Nibble on whole grain crackers both before and during the trip.

Nutrients That Help

☐ **Vitamin B$_6$** may help relieve nausea. Brewer's yeast is a rich natural source of this vitamin.

☐ **Vitamin C and vitamin K**, when taken together, are said to relieve morning sickness.

Beneficial Juices

☐ Ginger—was found in studies conducted at Brigham Young University to be more effective in preventing motion sickness than Dramamine, an over-the-counter motion-sickness pill. This study used ginger root powder in a capsule, but juicing the root and mixing it with another juice is cheaper and definitely more delicious. Ginger has been shown to be effective in treating motion sickness, seasickness, and morning sickness.

☐ Kale and spinach—sources of vitamin B_6.

☐ Sweet pepper, kale, and strawberry—sources of vitamin C.

☐ Turnip greens, broccoli, and lettuce—sources of vitamin K.

Suggested Juicing Recipes / Motion Sickness

Gingerberry Pops

1 quart blueberries
1-inch slice ginger root
1 medium bunch green
    grapes
3-oz. paper cups
Wooden popsicle sticks

Push blueberries and ginger through hopper with grapes. Pour juice into cups, add sticks, and freeze.

Ginger Tea

2-inch slice ginger root
¼ lemon
1 pint water
1 stick cinnamon, broken
4–5 cloves
Dash nutmeg or cardamom

Juice ginger and lemon. Place juice in saucepan, and add water, cinnamon, and cloves. Gently simmer. Add nutmeg or cardamom.

Ginger Hopper

¼-inch slice ginger root
4–5 carrots, greens removed
½ apple, seeded

*Push ginger through hopper
with carrots and apple.*

Ginger Fizz

¼-inch slice ginger root
1 apple, seeded
Sparkling water

*Push ginger through hopper
with apple. Pour juice into
ice-filled glass. Fill glass to
top with sparkling water.*

Ginger Ale

1 lemon wedge
¼-inch slice ginger root
1 medium bunch green
    grapes
Sparkling water

*Juice lemon. Push ginger
through hopper with grapes.
Pour juice into tall, ice-filled
glass. Fill glass to top with
sparkling water.*

K-Cooler

1 turnip green
1 stalk broccoli
1 red apple, seeded
Parsley sprig for garnish

*Juice vegetables and apple.
Pour juice into ice-filled glass,
and garnish with parsley.*

Strawberry Shake

1 pint strawberries
½ firm pear
1 ripe banana
1 Tbsp. brewer's yeast

*Push strawberries and pear
through hopper. Place juice,
banana, and yeast in blender
or food processor, and blend
until smooth.*

MUSCLE CRAMPS

Muscle cramps are painful, involuntary contractions caused by an imbalance of electrolytes (sodium, potassium, calcium, or magnesium), lack of water, or insufficient blood flow to the muscle. Cramps can be triggered by overexercise, very cold temperatures, dehydration, or any muscle irritation that causes pain. The pain impulse travels to the spinal cord, which responds by sending back impulses that create more pain, setting up a vicious cycle.

General Recommendations

Heat applied to the cramping muscle often brings fast relief. If you are prone to foot cramps at night, try wearing warm socks to bed or preheating the bed with a heating pad.

Dietary Modifications

1. *Follow the Basic Diet.* (See page 285.)

2. *Make it a practice to drink more water or juices.* Water is an essential nutrient we often forget about. Muscle cramping after exercise during hot weather is often due to dehydration. Whenever you sweat, drink plain water or one of the juice drinks recommended in this section. Always dilute fruit and vegetable juices with water when you drink them after exercising or when you are taking them to relieve cramps.

3. *Reduce or eliminate your consumption of all caffeine-containing beverages, such as coffee, tea, and some soft drinks.* These drinks can cause dehydration by increasing urine production.

Nutrients That Help

☐ **Sodium** helps control the chemical balance of the body.

☐ **Potassium** helps control the chemical balance of the body.

☐ **Calcium** helps control the chemical balance of the body.

☐ **Magnesium** helps control the chemical balance of the body.

☐ **Vitamin E** has relieved the pain of nighttime leg and foot cramps, rectal cramps, abdominal muscle cramps, and cramps following heavy exercise.

☐ **Vitamin C** helps to improve circulation.

☐ **B-complex vitamins** help to improve circulation. Ask your doctor about B-vitamin supplementation, as you will not be able to get sufficient amounts from juices.

Beneficial Juices

☐ Celery, carrot, and beet greens—good sources of sodium.

☐ Swiss chard, kale, and carrot—good sources of potassium.

☐ Kale, collard greens, and watercress—good sources of calcium.

☐ Collard greens and parsley—sources of magnesium.

☐ Asparagus, carrot, and spinach—sources of vitamin E.

☐ Red pepper, kale, and collard greens—sources of vitamin C.

Suggested Juicing Recipes / Muscle Cramps

Summertime Punch

1 large bunch green grapes
½ lime
2 stalks celery
Water

Juice grapes, lime, and celery. Mix juice with equal amount of water.

Mineral Tonic

Handful parsley
2 turnip leaves
1 kale leaf
4–5 carrots, greens removed

Roll up parsley in turnip and kale leaves, and push through hopper with carrots.

Summer Breeze

1 orange, peeled (leave white pithy part)
1 medium bunch green grapes
2 cups watermelon pieces, with rind
Mint sprig for garnish

Push orange, grapes, and watermelon through hopper. Pour juice into tall glass over crushed ice, and garnish with sprig of mint.

Sweet Magnesium Smoothie

1 pint blackberries
1 ripe banana
2 oz. silken tofu
1 Tbsp. brewer's yeast

Juice berries. Place juice, banana, tofu, and yeast in blender or food processor, and blend until smooth. Garnish with blackberries. Drink 1 hour before bedtime.

Magnesium Drink

1 garlic clove
Small handful parsley
4–5 carrots, greens removed
2 stalks celery
Parsley sprig for garnish

Wrap garlic in parsley, and push through hopper with carrots and celery. Pour juice into glass, and garnish with sprig of parsley.

Cucumber Cooler

1 tomato
1 cucumber
2 stalks celery
Parsley sprig for garnish

Juice tomato, pour juice into ice cube tray, and freeze. Juice cucumber and celery. Pour juice into tall glass, add tomato cubes, and garnish with sprig of parsley.

Mint Foam

1 handful mint
1 green apple, seeded
1 firm kiwi, peeled
Mint sprig for garnish

Bunch up mint and push through hopper with apple and kiwi. Pour juice into wine glass and garnish with sprig of mint.

NAUSEA

See MOTION SICKNESS.

OBESITY

See OVERWEIGHT/OBESITY.

OSTEOARTHRITIS

See ARTHRITIS.

OSTEOPOROSIS

Osteoporosis is a gradual loss of bone mass with a thinning of bone tissue and the appearance of small holes in the bone.

This condition can result in increased fractures, loss of height, pain in the hip and back, and curvature of the spine. Much of the publicity on osteoporosis has placed the blame on calcium deficiency, but calcium is only one component of bone. Non-dietary factors such as lack of exercise and estrogen deficiency also play important roles. It appears that calcium works best when combined with other treatments.

General Recommendations

Weight-bearing exercise, such as walking, is extremely important, since stress is necessary to lay down new bone. This is a true instance of "use it or lose it." Smoking may also affect calcium balance, so preserving calcium is yet another reason to quit smoking. Drugs such as isoniazid, corticosteroids, tetracycline, and thyroid preparations can also cause calcium loss, while antacids that contain aluminum can reduce calcium absorption.

Dietary Modifications

1. *Follow the Basic Diet.* (See page 285.) Its high fiber content may help prevent bone loss.

2. *Consider the possibility of hypoglycemia.* There is some evidence that individuals with osteoporosis may have glucose intolerance. (*See* HYPOGLYCEMIA in Part Two.)

3. *Avoid high-phosphate soft drinks such as colas and caffeine-containing beverages such as coffee and tea.* These drinks may increase calcium loss.

4. *Decrease the amount of salt you eat.* Salt increases calcium loss.

5. *Reduce your consumption of meat.* Some studies have indicated that a diet high in meat may promote osteoporosis. Eat meat at no more than one meal each day, and schedule several meatless days each week.

6. *Avoid drinking alcoholic beverages.* Alcohol, even in moderation, may increase the risk of hip fracture.

Nutrients That Help

☐ **Calcium** is the most abundant mineral in bone. There is much evidence to suggest that calcium intake in the teen years is extremely important. Many people cannot tolerate milk products and do not realize that vegetables such as kale and broccoli are high in calcium. The calcium in kale is absorbed just as well as, if not better than, the calcium in milk.

☐ **Magnesium**, like calcium, is found in bone and has a role in preventing bone loss.

☐ **Boron** is a trace mineral that is necessary to activate certain hormones that have a regulatory effect on bone deposition.

☐ **Vitamin K** enables the protein in bone to hold onto calcium molecules.

☐ **Vitamin D** is involved in bone mineral balance. This vitamin can be made by the body when the skin is exposed to sunlight. The best food source of vitamin D is cold-water fatty fish, like herring and tuna.

☐ **Anthocyanins and proanthocyanidins** are pigments that float within the cell sap. These compounds help the body to build strong collagen structures, and so may help stabilize bone structure.

Beneficial Juices

☐ Kale, collard greens, and parsley—excellent sources of calcium.

☐ Collard greens, parsley, and blackberry—sources of magnesium.

☐ Kale, collard greens, and turnip greens—sources of boron.

☐ Turnip greens, broccoli, lettuce, and cabbage—excellent sources of vitamin K.

☐ Red grape and blueberry—sources of anthocyanins.

Suggested Juicing Recipes / Osteoporosis

Calcium-Rich Cocktail

3 kale leaves
Small handful parsley
4–5 carrots, greens removed
½ apple, seeded

Bunch up kale and parsley, and push through hopper with carrots and apple.

K-Cooler

1 turnip green
1 stalk broccoli
1 red apple, seeded
Parsley sprig for garnish

Juice vegetables and apple. Pour juice into ice-filled glass, and garnish with parsley.

Magnesium Drink

1 garlic clove
Small handful parsley
4–5 carrots, greens removed
2 stalks celery
Parsley sprig for garnish

Wrap garlic in parsley, and push through hopper with carrots and celery. Pour juice into glass, and garnish with sprig of parsley.

Red Crush

1 medium bunch red grapes
½ cup cherries, pitted
½ cup blueberries
Handful whole berries (any
    kind)

Juice grapes, cherries, and berries. Pour juice into a glass or bowl over finely crushed ice. Spinkle whole berries on top, and eat with a spoon.

Sweet Calcium Shake

1 pint strawberries
6 oz. silken tofu

Juice strawberries. Place juice and tofu in blender or food processor, and blend until smooth. Garnish with strawberry.

Veggie Cocktail

Handful parsley
3 beet tops
2 stalks celery
4 carrots, greens removed

*Bunch up parsley and beet
tops, and push through
hopper with celery and
carrots.*

Sweet and Sour Cherry Cream
---

1 cup cherries, pitted
4 oz. nonfat yogurt

*Juice cherries. Place juice and
yogurt in blender or food
processor, and blend until
smooth.*

OVERWEIGHT/OBESITY

Obesity is an excess of body fat. Anyone who is 20 percent
over the norm for his or her age, build, and height is considered obese. This is a three-sided problem. Lack of exercise,
poor nutrition, and emotional difficulties all contribute to
obesity. To lose weight permanently, the overweight individual
must address all three areas. Rather than focusing on losing
pounds, focus on improving your eating habits and building
fitness. Not many of us are genetically programmed to look like
Barbie or He Man dolls. Make peace with the shape you are.

General Recommendations

Don't spend money on highly advertised diet programs. Invest
instead in a good counselor who specializes in weight problems
and a membership in a health club that caters to people who
share your desire to lose weight. Forget about counting
calories, and concentrate on getting the junk out of your diet
and the lead out of your feet. Start by walking thirty minutes
each day. Also, read the book *Diets Don't Work* by Bob
Schwartz.

Dietary Modifications

1. *Follow the Basic Diet*. (See page 285.) Read *The Goldbeck's Guide to Good Food* by Nikki and David Goldbeck and *The New American Diet* by Sonja and William Connor (see the Suggested Reading List on page 323) for guidance in setting up a kitchen and developing recipes.

2. *After you have accustomed yourself to this healthy way of eating, start to keep a food diary*. In a notebook, write down everything you eat, when you eat it, the amounts consumed (very important), and how you feel when you eat. For the first three days, measure everything that goes into your mouth in order to develop a sense of proportion. Overweight individuals have a tendency to underestimate portion size. After two weeks, review your diary to see if there are any times of day, feelings, or stressful events that are associated with overeating.

3. *Gradually start to reduce your portion size*. Together with your exercise program, this should result in weight loss. You should never try to lose more than one to two pounds a week since large weight losses mean a loss of muscle as well.

4. *Be sure to dilute your fruit juices to reduce calories*. Nourish your body with vegetable juices instead.

Suggested Juicing Recipes / Overweight/Obesity

Super-Eight Stress Reliever

---

1 kale leaf
1 collard leaf
Small handful parsley
1 stalk celery
1 carrot, greens removed
½ red pepper
1 tomato
1 broccoli floweret
Celery stalk for garnish

Bunch up leaves and parsley, and push through hopper with celery and carrot. Follow with red pepper, tomato, and broccoli. Garnish with celery stalk.

Warm Apple Pie

1 tart apple, seeded	*Juice apple. In small pan,*
Water	*bring 2 oz. juice and 4 oz.*
Apple pie spice	*water to boil. Season with*
Cinnamon stick for garnish	*liberal amount of spice. Serve*
	in teacup. Garnish with
	cinnamon stick.

Low-Sugar Pop

1 apple, seeded	*Juice apple and lime. Pour*
¼ lime	*juice into tall, ice-filled glass.*
Sparkling water	*Fill glass to top with*
	sparkling water.

Cucumber Cooler

1 tomato	*Juice tomato, pour juice into*
1 cucumber	*ice cube tray, and freeze.*
2 stalks celery	*Juice cucumber and celery.*
Parsley sprig for garnish	*Pour juice into tall glass, add*
	tomato cubes, and garnish
	with sprig of parsley.

Cherie's Cleansing Cocktail

¼-inch slice ginger root	*Push ginger, beet, and apple*
1 beet	*through hopper with carrots.*
½ apple, seeded	
4 carrots, greens removed	

Mineral Tonic

Handful parsley	*Roll up parsley in turnip and*
2 turnip leaves	*kale leaves, and push*
1 kale leaf	*through hopper with carrots.*
4–5 carrots, greens removed	

Harvest Soup

2–3 garlic cloves
1 kale leaf
1 large tomato
2 stalks celery
1 collard leaf, chopped
1 Tbsp. croutons

Roll garlic in kale leaf, and push through hopper with tomato and celery. Place juice in saucepan, add chopped collards, and gently heat. Garnish with croutons.

PERIODONTAL DISEASE

Gingivitis is an inflammation of the gums. It is considered to be an early stage of periodontal disease caused by a buildup of plaque on the teeth. It is believed that the accumulated plaque causes the gums to become infected and swollen. If left untreated, gingivitis can progress to periodontitis, a condition in which the inflammation spreads to the bone. Periodontitis (also called pyorrhea) is a major cause of tooth loss in adults and can result from poor dental hygiene, poor nutrition, overconsumption of sugars, excess alcohol consumption, drugs, and smoking. This condition must be treated by a dentist. The role of nutrition is to strengthen the tissues and build defense mechanisms that prevent bacterial toxins from penetrating the gums.

General Recommendations

Besides a sound diet, good dental hygiene is your best weapon against periodontal disease. Use dental floss daily to clean and stimulate the gums, and brush your teeth after every meal, using a soft toothbrush on both the teeth and the gums.

Once periodontal disease begins, it must be treated by a dentist. If you suspect periodontal disease, see your doctor and then try some of the remedies below.

Dietary Modifications

1. **Follow the Immune Support Diet.** (See page 293.)

2. Eat a high-fiber diet. This will increase salivary secretions, which may have a protective effect.

3. Eliminate simple sugars. Sugar inhibits the function of white blood cells. Sugar also promotes tooth decay.

4. Reduce your consumption of fruit juices other than those made of berries.

5. *See also* INFECTIONS in Part Two.

Nutrients That Help

☐ **Beta-carotene and zinc** work together. Vitamin A is necessary for tissue synthesis and zinc is necessary for wound healing. Beta-carotene is the preferred form of vitamin A because of its antioxidant properties and lack of toxicity.

☐ **Vitamin C** strengthens the immune system and decreases the permeability of gingival cells.

☐ **Bioflavonoids** are the most important compounds in the treatment of periodontal disease. They are extremely effective in reducing inflammation and stabilizing collagen structures. (Collagen forms connective tissue.)

☐ **Folic acid** reduces the inflammation of gingival tissues.

Beneficial Juices

☐ Kale, parsley, and collard greens—low-sugar sources of beta-carotene.

☐ Parsley and garlic—sources of zinc.

☐ Kale, parsley, and collard greens—low-sugar sources of vitamin C.

☐ Blueberry, cabbage, and tomato—sources of bioflavonoids.

☐ Spinach, kale, and beet greens—sources of folic acid.

☐ Ginger—a natural anti-inflammatory agent.

☐ Pineapple—a natural anti-inflammatory agent.

Suggested Juicing Recipes / Periodontal Disease

Hot Tomato on Ice

1 tomato
1 red pepper
Dash hot pepper sauce
4 lettuce leaves
1 stalk broccoli
Parsley sprig for garnish

Juice tomato and red pepper, add dash of pepper sauce, pour into ice cube tray, and freeze. Juice lettuce and broccoli. Pour juice into tall glass, add tomato cubes, and garnish with sprig of parsley.

Harvest Soup

2–3 garlic cloves
1 kale leaf
1 large tomato
2 stalks celery
1 collard leaf, chopped
1 Tbsp. croutons

Roll garlic in kale leaf, and push through hopper with tomato and celery. Place juice in saucepan, add chopped collards, and gently heat. Garnish with croutons.

Bluemint Fizz

Handful mint
1 pint blueberries
Sparkling water
Mint sprig for garnish

Bunch up mint and push through hopper with berries. Pour juice into tall, ice-filled glass. Fill glass to top with sparkling water. Garnish with sprig of mint.

Mineral Tonic

Handful parsley
2 turnip leaves
1 kale leaf
4–5 carrots, greens removed

Roll up parsley in turnip and kale leaves, and push through hopper with carrots.

Ginger Hopper

¼-inch slice ginger root
4–5 carrots, greens removed
½ apple, seeded

*Push ginger through hopper
with carrots and apple.*

PREMENSTRUAL SYNDROME

Premenstrual syndrome (PMS) is a condition characterized by recurrent symptoms that develop during the seven to fourteen days prior to menstruation. More than 150 symptoms have been noted, ranging from emotional difficulties such as nervousness, mood swings, and depression to gastrointestinal problems such as bloating, sugar cravings, and constipation. Headaches, backaches, water retention, fatigue, joint pain, and breast swelling and tenderness are also common complaints. This syndrome is caused by a combination of physical, psychological, and nutritional factors, and a complete discussion of PMS is beyond the scope of this work. For more information, read the *Encyclopedia of Natural Medicine* by Michael Murray and Joseph Pizzorno.

General Recommendations

In some cases, exercise provides great benefits, easing cramps and lightening depression. Sometimes, hypoglycemia is the underlying problem. If you suspect that this may be true for you, see your doctor. (*See* HYPOGLYCEMIA in Part Two.) For many women, a change of diet reduces the severity of or totally eliminates symptoms.

Dietary Modifications

1. Follow the Sugar Metabolism Disorder Diet. (See page 288.) The risk for PMS increases when a woman's diet is nutritionally poor. Chronic dieting depletes the body of the nutrients necessary for normal reproductive functioning.

2. *Limit your consumption of refined carbohydrates such as sugar, honey, and white flour.* Fruit juices should be limited to pineapple juice, which contains a muscle relaxant, and watermelon and grapes, which are natural diuretics (i.e., they relieve water retention).

3. *Restrict your consumption of alcohol, tobacco, and salt.* Alcohol and tobacco inhibit factors that decrease inflammation. Salt increases fluid retention.

4. *Restrict your intake of methylxanthines found in coffee, tea, and chocolate.* These substances have been linked with fibrocystic breast disease, which is one cause of breast tenderness.

5. *Avoid caffeine-containing beverages such as coffee, tea, and colas.* Caffeine may cause breast tenderness in some women.

6. *See also* MENSTRUAL PROBLEMS and WATER RETENTION in Part Two.

Nutrients That Help

☐ **Beta-carotene**, which is converted to vitamin A in the body, has been shown to be effective in reducing PMS symptoms when taken during the second half of the menstrual cycle.

☐ **Magnesium** deficiency may cause PMS symptoms in some women.

☐ **Bromelain** is thought to be a smooth-muscle relaxant.

☐ **Vitamin E** is one of the healing nutrients, and can reduce breast tenderness. See your doctor regarding vitamin E supplementation.

☐ **Vitamin B$_6$ and riboflavin** may reduce PMS symptoms. They should be taken together, since a deficiency of riboflavin can interfere with the use of vitamin B$_6$.

Beneficial Juices

☐ Beet greens, Swiss chard, and collard greens—good sources of beta-carotene.

☐ Collard greens and parsley—sources of magnesium.

☐ Pineapple—fresh juice is a source of bromelain.

☐ Kale, turnip greens, and red pepper—good sources of vitamin B6.

☐ Collard greens, kale, and parsley—good sources of riboflavin.

☐ Watermelon, cucumber, grape, and lettuce—traditional, natural diuretics.

Suggested Juicing Recipes / Premenstrual Syndrome

Tossed Salad

1 kale leaf	Bunch up the leaves and
1 turnip leaf	spinach, and push through
Handful spinach	hopper with tomatoes.
2 tomatoes	Garnish with cherry tomato.
1 cherry tomato for garnish	

Bromelain Special

| ¼ pineapple, with skin | Push pineapple through |
| | hopper. |

Orange Spice Tea

½-inch ginger root	Push ginger and orange
1 orange, peeled (leave white	through hopper. Pour 2 oz. of
pithy part)	juice into teacup and fill with
Water	boiling water. Garnish with
Cinnamon stick for garnish	cinnamon stick.

Mineral Tonic

Handful parsley
2 turnip leaves
1 kale leaf
4–5 carrots, greens removed

Roll up parsley in turnip and kale leaves, and push through hopper with carrots.

Watermelon Juice

2-inch slice watermelon, with rind
Orange slice for garnish

Juice watermelon. Pour juice into glass and garnish with orange slice.

Magnesium Drink

1 garlic clove
Small handful parsley
4–5 carrots, greens removed
2 stalks celery
Parsley sprig for garnish

Wrap garlic in parsley, and push through hopper with carrots and celery. Pour juice into glass, and garnish with sprig of parsley.

Pineapple Protein Shake

3 pineapple rings, with skin
4 oz. soymilk
1 ripe banana
2–3 Tbsp. protein powder
Pineapple spear for garnish

Juice pineapple. Place juice, soymilk, banana, and protein powder into blender or food processor, and blend until smooth. Pour juice into tall glass and garnish with pineapple spear.

PROSTATE ENLARGEMENT

The prostate is a donut-shaped male sex gland the size of a chestnut. It sits at the neck of the bladder and surrounds the urethra, the narrow tube through which sperm and urine both flow. The prostate secretes the milky white fluid that transports and protects the sperm. Nearly 60 percent of men over forty years of age have an enlargement of this gland (called benign prostatic hypertrophy), which slowly begins to strangle the urethra, causing symptoms of increased need to urinate and decreased flow and force of urine. If left untreated, the growing gland will eventually cut off all flow of urine. The usual treatment is surgery.

General Recommendations

The cause of benign prostatic hypertrophy appears to be decreasing hormone levels. Stress can further affect these levels, and so stress reduction techniques may be helpful. Sitz baths can bring temporary relief.

Dietary Modifications

1. Follow the Basic Diet. (See page 285.)

2. Eliminate beer from your diet. Beer can increase levels of prolactin, a pituitary hormone. Reduced prolactin levels usually mean a decrease in symptoms.

3. Decrease serum cholesterol levels. One study indicated that cholesterol can inhibit the breakdown of prostate cells, possibly resulting in prostate enlargement. (*See* CHOLES-TEROLEMIA in Part Two.)

4. Eat a whole-foods diet. As the amount of toxins in our environment has increased, so has the incidence of prostate enlargement. Whole foods contain vitamins, minerals, fiber, and anutrients that are natural detoxifiers.

5. Add high-zinc foods such as pumpkin seeds, pecans, split peas, whole grains, and lima beans to your diet. Zinc has been shown to reduce the size of the prostate and lessen symptoms in some men. In addition, zinc deficiency has been linked with cancer of the prostate.

Nutrients That Help

☐ **Zinc** reduces the size of the prostate and lessens symptoms in some individuals. Pumpkin seeds are exceptional sources of both zinc and the essential fatty acids (EFAs).

☐ **Essential fatty acids (EFAs)** deficiency has been linked with prostate enlargement. Try taking two teaspoons of flaxseed (linseed) oil per day. (Essential fatty acids cannot be obtained from juices.)

☐ **Vitamin B₆** is involved with hormone metabolism and works with zinc to reduce prolactin levels.

Beneficial Juices

☐ Ginger, parsley, and carrot—sources of zinc.

☐ Kale, spinach, and turnip greens—sources of vitamin B₆.

Suggested Juicing Recipes / Prostate Enlargement

Tossed Salad

1 kale leaf
1 turnip leaf
Handful spinach
2 tomatoes
1 cherry tomato for garnish

Bunch up the leaves and spinach, and push through hopper with tomatoes. Garnish with cherry tomato.

Strawberry Shake

1 pint strawberries
½ firm pear
1 ripe banana
1 Tbsp. brewer's yeast

Push strawberries and pear through hopper. Place juice, banana, and yeast in blender or food processor, and blend until smooth.

Ginger Hopper

¼-inch slice ginger root
4–5 carrots, greens removed
½ apple, seeded

*Push ginger through hopper
with carrots and apple.*

Energy Shake

Handful parsley
4–6 carrots, greens removed
Parsley sprig for garnish

*Bunch up parsley and push
through hopper with carrots.
Garnish with sprig of parsley.*

Ginger Ale

1 lemon wedge
¼-inch slice ginger root
1 medium bunch green
    grapes
Sparkling water

*Juice lemon. Push ginger
through hopper with grapes.
Pour juice into tall, ice-filled
glass. Fill glass to top with
sparkling water.*

PSORIASIS

This skin disease results when skin cells divide too quickly—
up to 1,000 times faster than normal. The result is a pile-up
of skin in the form of itchy silvery scales on the buttocks, scalp,
and soles of the feet and on the backs of the wrists, elbows,
knees, and ankles. In addition, toenails and fingernails may
lose their luster and develop pits and ridges. An outbreak can
be triggered by stress, infection, illness, surgery, sunburn,
viral or bacterial infections, or drugs like lithium. Psoriasis is
most common between the ages of fifteen and twenty-five. This
disorder is not infectious, and presently there is no cure.
Treatment consists of increasing compounds that cause skin
cells to mature and decreasing compounds such as
polyamines, which may increase cell overgrowth.

General Recommendations

Expose the affected area to sunlight for one hour each day. The application of heating pads has also proved to be effective. Both sunlight and heating pads may help to reduce the severity of symptoms.

Dietary Modifications

1. *Follow the Basic Diet.* (See page 285.) Poor dietary habits are linked with susceptibility to skin diseases.

2. *Rule out the possibility of food allergies.* To identify allergies to food, try the Elimination Diet. (See page 296.)

3. *Eat a diet high in fiber.* Fiber helps bind toxins in the bowel that increase the rate of skin cell growth. At each meal, over half the food on your plate should be raw.

4. *Detoxify the bowel with a cleansing fast.* (See the Cleansing Diets on page 299.)

5. *Eliminate alcohol.* Studies have shown that alcohol worsens the symptoms of psoriasis.

6. *Eat more mackerel, salmon, and herring.* Cold-water fatty fish contain fish oils that slow or halt skin inflammation.

Nutrients That Help

☐ **Zinc** losses through skin shedding are greater in psoriasis. Zinc is also necessary for the absorption of linoleic acid, a fatty acid necessary for healthy skin. Pumpkin seeds are an excellent source of both zinc and linoleic acid.

☐ **Selenium** helps decrease the formation of inflammatory compounds.

☐ **Folic acid** may be deficient in psoriatic skin.

☐ **Beta-carotene**, which the body converts into vitamin A, decreases the polyamines, substances that are implicated in accelerating skin growth.

Beneficial Juices

☐ Parsley and carrot—sources of zinc.

☐ Red Swiss chard, garlic, and orange—sources of selenium.

☐ Spinach, kale, and beet greens—good sources of folic acid.

☐ Carrot, kale, and cantaloupe—excellent sources of beta-carotene.

☐ Beet—a potent detoxifier.

☐ Pineapple—contains the enzyme bromelain, which aids in protein digestion, decreasing polyamines.

☐ Papaya—the papaya contains the enzyme papain, which aids in protein digestion, decreasing polyamines.

☐ Ginger—a natural anti-inflammatory agent.

Suggested Juicing Recipes / Psoriasis

Cherie's Cleansing Cocktail

¼-inch slice ginger root
1 beet
½ apple, seeded
4 carrots, greens removed

Push ginger, beet, and apple through hopper with carrots.

Mineral Tonic

Handful parsley
2 turnip leaves
1 kale leaf
4–5 carrots, greens removed

Roll up parsley in turnip and kale leaves, and push through hopper with carrots.

Tropical Squeeze

1 firm papaya, peeled
¼-inch slice ginger root
1 pear

Juice papaya. Push ginger through hopper with pear.

Maureen's Spicy Tonic

¼ pineapple, with skin
½ apple, seeded
¼-inch slice ginger root

Push pineapple through hopper with apple and ginger.

Body Cleanser

½ cucumber
1 beet
½ apple, seeded
4 carrots, greens removed

Push cucumber, beet, and apple through hopper with carrots.

Spiced Orange Foam

¼-inch slice ginger root
2 large oranges, peeled (leave white pithy part)
½ apple, seeded
Orange twist for garnish

Push ginger through hopper with orange and apple. Serve with twist of orange.

Garden Salad Special

3 broccoli flowerets
1 garlic clove
4–5 carrots or 2 tomatoes
2 stalks celery
½ green pepper

Push broccoli and garlic through hopper with carrots or tomatoes. Follow with celery and green pepper.

RAYNAUD'S DISEASE

See CIRCULATION PROBLEMS.

RHEUMATOID ARTHRITIS

See ARTHRITIS.

SENILITY

See ALZHEIMER'S DISEASE.

SKIN DISORDERS

See ACNE; AGE SPOTS; ECZEMA; PSORIASIS.

SORE THROAT

Many sore throats are the result of bacteria or viruses invading the tissues lining the throat. A battle takes place between the invading army of germs and your body's immune system. The result of this battle is inflammation, which causes swelling and pain. Your physician may recommend antibiotics, which work by killing attacking bacteria. Over-the-counter drugs work by masking the symptoms. The natural remedies below work by making your immune system stronger so that it can protect your cells from infection more effectively.

Some sore throats are caused not by infection, but by other irritants, including dust, smoke, fumes, extremely hot foods or drinks, or allergens such as pollen. Just like invading bacteria, these irritants cause the throat to be inflamed and painful. Although most of the suggestions provided below are aimed at bacterial or viral infections, those suggestions that address the problem of inflammation will help to soothe your sore throat regardless of the cause. If you suspect that allergies are the culprit, see your doctor.

General Recommendations

Slow down and rest in bed if at all possible. If the pain persists or you suspect a strep infection, contact your doctor. It is best to treat a strep throat with antibiotics. (For more information, see INFECTIONS in Part Two.) Remember that if you are taking antibiotics for any reason, you should also take an acidophilus source such as yogurt.

Dietary Modifications

1. *Follow the Immune Support Diet.* (See page 293.)

2. *Lower your consumption of simple sugars, including fruit juices.* Sugar weakens the ability of white blood cells to destroy bacteria.

3. *Drink large amounts of fluids, such as diluted vegetable juices and broths.* For those over seventeen years of age, a Juice Fast for the first one or two days would be beneficial. (See page 301.)

4. *Increase your consumption of garlic, a natural antibiotic.* The allicin component of garlic is an effective killer of streptococcal bacteria.

5. *Add ginger to your diet.* Ginger is a natural anti-inflammatory agent.

6. *Sip fresh pineapple juice.* Bromelain, an enzyme present only in raw pineapple, has been found to reduce inflammation and swelling. Pineapple is considered a traditional remedy for sore throat.

7. *See also* COMMON COLD in Part Two.

Nutrients That Help

☐ **Bromelain** reduces inflammation and swelling.

□ **Vitamin C and bioflavonoids** are immune system strengtheners that help your body fight infection.

□ **Beta-carotene** supports the immune system.

Beneficial Juices

□ Pineapple—the only source of bromelain, an anti-inflammatory agent.

□ Kale, broccoli, and red pepper—low-sugar sources of vitamin C.

□ Cabbage and tomato—low-sugar sources of bioflavonoids.

□ Carrot, collard greens, and kale—sources of beta-carotene.

□ Garlic—a natural antibiotic.

□ Ginger—a natural anti-inflammatory agent.

Suggested Juicing Recipes / Sore Throat

Tahitian Gargle

1 whole lemon

Juice lemon. Gargle with juice full-strength.

Hot Soother

½ lemon
1 tsp. honey (do not use for
　children under 1 year old)
Hot water

Juice lemon, add honey, and mix with hot water in a mug. Sip slowly.

Soothing Pops

3 pineapple rings, with skin
¼-inch slice ginger root
1 firm pear
3-oz. paper cups
Wooden popsicle sticks

Juice pineapple. Push ginger through hopper with pear. Pour juice into cups, add sticks, and freeze.

Instant Soup

2–3 garlic cloves
1 bunch spinach
½ cucumber
1 stalk celery
2 Tbsp. finely chopped
    spinach and celery
Parsley sprig for garnish

Wrap garlic cloves in spinach,
and push through hopper
with cucumber and celery.
Place juice in pan, add
chopped vegetables, and
gently heat. Garnish with
sprig of parsley. Serve hot.

Immune Builder

Handful parsley
1 garlic clove
5 carrots, greens removed
3 stalks celery

Bunch up parsley, and push
through hopper with garlic,
carrots, and celery.

Spiced Mint Tea

1 bunch mint
½-inch slice ginger root
1 orange, peeled (leave white
    pithy part)
Water

Bunch up mint and push
through hopper with ginger
and orange. Put 2 oz. juice
into teacup and add 4 oz.
boiling water.

Maureen's Spicy Tonic

¼ pineapple, with skin
½ apple, seeded
¼-inch slice ginger root

Push pineapple through
hopper with apple and ginger.

Ginger Roger

3 pineapple rings, with skin
¼-inch slice ginger root

Push pineapple slices and
ginger through hopper.

SPASTIC COLON

See COLITIS.

STRESS

Stress has been called the wear and tear of life. It can be caused by many things: financial problems, illness, relationships, a high-pressure job, and loneliness. Stress is a highly personal reaction. Something that invigorates one person may stress another. This disorder causes fight-or-flight hormones to flood the body, and if the stress is prolonged, it can cause decreased energy, impaired resistance to infection, and a host of physical complaints such as headaches, gastrointestinal problems, high blood pressure, dizziness, and loss of appetite. Treatment consists of identifying and reducing the triggers of stress and replenishing the nutrients expended in the stress response.

General Recommendations

Take the time to identify the major sources of stress in your life, and discover coping mechanisms for the stresses you cannot avoid. Practice relaxation techniques, get a good night's sleep, and get into the habit of deep breathing. Physical exercise in the form of walking is also a great stress reliever. Hobbies, too, can be good outlets for pent-up energies resulting from stress.

Dietary Modifications

1. *Follow the Immune Support Diet.* (See page 293.) A good diet can go a long way in helping your body deal with stress.

2. Increase your consumption of fiber. Stress increases cholesterol levels; fiber decreases cholesterol absorption.

3. Decrease your consumption of sugar. Sugar puts more stress on your immune system by depleting chromium and depressing white blood cell action.

4. Increase your consumption of foods that thin the blood, such as ginger, garlic, and cantaloupe. The stress reaction thickens the blood, leaving the body more susceptible to heart attack or stroke.

5. Avoid caffeine, alcohol, and drugs. Although these substances may offer temporary relief, in the long run, they can actually make stress worse.

Nutrients That Help

☐ **Pantothenic acid** is lost during the stress reaction and must be replenished.

☐ **Vitamin C** is lost during the stress reaction and must be replenished. This nutrient is also an antioxidant, and so helps protect the body during stress reactions.

☐ **Zinc** is lost during the stress reaction and must be replenished.

☐ **Magnesium** is lost during the stress reaction and must be replenished.

☐ **Potassium** is lost during the stress reaction and must be replenished.

☐ **Chromium** is lost during the stress reaction and must be replenished. Brewer's yeast is a good source of chromium.

☐ **Beta-carotene** is an antioxidant, and so helps protect the body during stress reactions.

☐ **B-complex vitamins** are known as antistress vitamins. See your doctor about B-vitamin supplements.

Beneficial Juices

☐ Broccoli and kale—sources of pantothenic acid.

☐ Red pepper, kale, and collard greens—sources of vitamin C.

☐ Ginger, parsley, and carrot—sources of zinc.

☐ Collard greens and parsley—excellent sources of magnesium.

☐ Parsley, Swiss chard, and spinach—sources of potassium.

☐ Carrot, collard greens, and parsley—excellent sources of beta-carotene.

☐ Garlic, cantaloupe, and ginger—sources of blood-thinning compounds.

Suggested Juicing Recipes / Stress

Ginger Hopper

¼-inch slice ginger root
4–5 carrots, greens removed
½ apple, seeded

Push ginger through hopper with carrots and apple.

Magnesium Drink

1 garlic clove
Small handful parsley
4–5 carrots, greens removed
2 stalks celery
Parsley sprig for garnish

Wrap garlic in parsley, and push through hopper with carrots and celery. Pour juice into glass, and garnish with sprig of parsley.

Strawberry Shake

1 pint strawberries
½ firm pear
1 ripe banana
1 Tbsp. brewer's yeast

Push strawberries and pear through hopper. Place juice, banana, and yeast in blender or food processor, and blend until smooth.

Spicy Cantaloupe Shake

¼-inch slice ginger root
½ cantaloupe, with skin

*Push ginger through hopper
with cantaloupe.*

Super-Eight Stress Reliever

1 kale leaf
1 collard leaf
Small handful parsley
1 stalk celery
1 carrot, greens removed
½ red pepper
1 tomato
1 broccoli floweret
Celery stalk for garnish

*Bunch up leaves and parsley,
and push through hopper
with celery and carrot. Follow
with red pepper, tomato, and
broccoli. Garnish with celery
stalk.*

Garlic Express

Handful parsley
1 garlic clove
4–5 carrots, greens removed
2 stalks celery

*Bunch up parsley and push
through hopper with garlic,
carrots, and celery.*

Traditional Sleep Potion

3–4 lettuce leaves
1 stalk celery

*Bunch up lettuce and push
through hopper with celery.
Drink 30 minutes before
bedtime.*

Potassium Broth

Handful parsley
Handful spinach
4–5 carrots, greens removed
2 stalks celery

*Bunch up parsley and
spinach leaves, and push
through hopper with carrots
and celery.*

Surgery Preparation

How quickly your body is able to repair itself is directly related to how well nourished it is. Proper nourishment is particularly important when surgery is planned. The outcome and length of recovery can be improved when your body is prepared for the stresses of surgery. The suggestions below will help prevent infection by boosting your immune system and supplying your body with the nutrients necessary to rebuild injured tissues. If you've already undergone surgery and are now recuperating, these tips will be just as valuable.

General Recommendations

When you pack your bag for the hospital, be sure to include your juicer! Make arrangements with your doctor and the hospital ahead of time, and have a friend or relative juice for you in your room.

Dietary Modifications

1. Follow the Immune Support Diet. (See page 293.)

2. Make sure you get generous amounts of protein before and after surgery. Protein is the basic building block of cells.

3. Eat a variety of dark, leafy greens. These vegetables are sources of vitamin K, needed for proper blood clotting, and iron, needed to support the immune system.

4. Garlic and ginger are natural blood thinners, and should be used sparingly before surgery. After you come home, garlic can be used generously as a natural antibiotic, and ginger can be used as a natural anti–inflammatory agent.

5. Add pineapple juice to your diet. This juice contains the enzyme bromelain, which helps to reduce swelling in the mouth after dental surgery. Pineapple juice may also help to reduce inflammation elsewhere in the body.

6. *See also* INFECTIONS and INFLAMMATION in Part Two.

Nutrients That Help

☐ **Beta-carotene** is a healing nutrient.

☐ **Vitamin E** is a healing nutrient. Speak to your doctor about supplementation in therapeutic amounts.

☐ **Zinc** is a healing nutrient. Speak to your doctor about supplementation in therapeutic amounts.

☐ **Vitamin C,** an antioxidant, promotes new tissue formation.

☐ **Vitamin K** is necessary for proper blood clotting.

☐ **Iron** is needed to help support the immune system.

☐ **Bromelain** helps to reduce swelling.

Beneficial Juices

☐ Kale, carrot, cantaloupe, and parsley—high in beta-carotene.

☐ Kale, red pepper, and strawberry—high in vitamin C.

☐ Turnip greens, broccoli, and lettuce—high in vitamin K.

☐ Parsley and kale—high in iron.

☐ Pineapple—a source of bromelain if made fresh.

☐ Garlic—a natural antibiotic. This can be used generously after surgery. Before surgery, however, it should be used only sparingly, as garlic is a natural blood thinner.

☐ Ginger—a natural anti-inflammatory agent. This juice can be used generously after surgery. Before surgery, however, it should be used only sparingly, as ginger is a natural blood thinner.

Suggested Juicing Recipes /
Surgery Preparation

Hawaiian Ice

½ pineapple, with skin
¼-inch slice ginger root
1 apple, seeded
3-oz. paper cups
Wooden popsicle sticks

Juice fruit, pour into cups,
add sticks, and freeze. Good
for those who have just had
dental surgery.

Hot Tomato on Ice

1 tomato
1 red pepper
Dash hot pepper sauce
4 lettuce leaves
1 stalk broccoli
Parsley sprig for garnish

Juice tomato and red pepper,
add dash of pepper sauce,
pour into ice cube tray, and
freeze. Juice lettuce and
broccoli. Pour juice into tall
glass, add tomato cubes, and
garnish with sprig of parsley.

Garlic Express

Handful parsley
1 garlic clove
4–5 carrots, greens removed
2 stalks celery

Bunch up parsley and push
through hopper with garlic,
carrots, and celery.

Ginger Hopper

¼-inch slice ginger root
4–5 carrots, greens removed
½ apple, seeded

Push ginger through hopper
with carrots and apple.

K-Cooler

1 turnip green
1 stalk broccoli
1 red apple, seeded
Parsley sprig for garnish

Juice vegetables and apple.
Pour juice into ice-filled glass,
and garnish with parsley.

Blood Enricher

1 turnip leaf
1 kale leaf
Handful parsley
4–5 carrots, greens removed

Bunch up leaves and parsley, and push through hopper with carrots. High in vitamin C and iron. Drink daily a week or two before surgery.

THROMBOSIS

Thrombosis is an abnormal condition in which a blood clot develops within a blood vessel of the body. This clotting can be brought on by the formation of cholesterol-containing masses known as plaques in the walls of blood vessels. Plaques present a rough surface that causes platelets to adhere and form clots. Known as a thrombus, the clot may damage tissues by cutting off blood supply. If the thrombus is dislodged, it can travel to smaller blood vessels where the thrombus, now called an embolus, can block circulation to vital organs. Blood clots can cause such conditions as myocardial infarction (heart attack), pulmonary embolus (the lodging of a blood clot in the lungs), and thrombophlebitis (the inflammation of a vein, often accompanied by the formation of a clot).

Even in a healthy body, occasional rough places appear on vessel walls. It is believed that blood clotting is a continuous process inside the body and is continually controlled by clot-preventing and clot-dissolving mechanisms through substances know as anticoagulants. Anticoagulants prevent the conversion of the blood plasma protein prothrombin to thrombin, an enzyme that is essential in the formation of clots.

General Recommendations

If you have a blood clot, a doctor's care is necessary. The following dietary recommendations should also be observed to prevent further clots from forming. As with any condition, prevention is the best cure.

Dietary Modifications

1. *Follow the Basic Diet.* (See page 285.)

2. *Avoid saturated fats.* Saturated fat is closely related to the clotting activity of platelets and their response to thrombin, the substance that forms clots. Fat raises the level of fibrinogen, a clot-promoting substance. Saturated fat is found in animal products such as red meat and dairy products, and in certain vegetable fats, such as coconut oil. Avoid margarine. We suggest using Better Butter as a spread. Soften one pound of butter in your blender, add one cup of cold-pressed or expeller-pressed oil, like safflower or sunflower oil, blend, and refrigerate.

3. *Avoid sugar.* Use only natural sweeteners such as honey, pure maple sugar, or fruit juice concentrates, and restrict your intake of these sweeteners to no more than 10 percent of your diet. Sugar is associated with increased platelet adhesiveness.

4. *Consume generous amounts of those foods that act as anticoagulants, including chili pepper, garlic, onion, eggplant, olive oil, ginger root, melon, and pineapple.* Cold-water fatty fish, fish oils, and flaxseed (linseed) oil (buy only those oils that are stored in opaque bottles and refrigerated) are good sources of omega-3 fatty acids and are good anticoagulants as well.

5. *Include omega-6 fatty acids in your diet by taking evening primrose oil, one of the best sources of gamma linoleic acid, the most active omega-6 fatty acid.* Omega-6 fatty acids have been shown to minimize the formation of blood clots.

Nutrients That Help

☐ **Vitamin B6** may inhibit platelet adhesiveness and prolong clotting time.

☐ **Vitamin C** may decrease platelet adhesiveness.

☐ **Vitamin E** may inhibit platelet adhesiveness.

☐ **Calcium** may inhibit platelet adhesiveness.

☐ **Magnesium** may inhibit platelet adhesiveness.

☐ **Selenium** may reduce platelet adhesiveness.

☐ **Bromelain** is said to inhibit platelet adhesiveness.

Beneficial Juices

☐ Kale, spinach, turnip greens, and green pepper—sources of vitamin B6.

☐ Kale, parsley, green pepper, and spinach—sources of vitamin C.

☐ Spinach, asparagus, and carrot—sources of vitamin E.

☐ Kale, parsley, watercress, and beet greens—sources of calcium.

☐ Beet greens, spinach, parsley, and garlic—sources of magnesium.

☐ Turnip, garlic, and orange—sources of selenium.

☐ Pineapple—the only source of bromelain.

Suggested Juicing Recipes / Thrombosis

Bromelain Special

¼ pineapple, with skin

Push pineapple through hopper.

Monkey Shake

½ orange, peeled (leave white pithy part)
½ papaya, peeled
1 banana
Orange twist for garnish

Push orange through hopper with papaya. Place juice and banana in blender or food processor, and blend until smooth. Garnish with orange twist.

Cantaloupe Shake

½ cantaloupe, with skin   *Cut cantaloupe in strips, and*
                                 push through hopper.

Garden Salad Special

3 broccoli flowerets   *Push broccoli and garlic*
1 garlic clove   *through hopper with carrots*
4–5 carrots or 2 tomatoes   *or tomatoes. Follow with*
2 stalks celery   *celery and green pepper.*
½ green pepper

Spring Tonic

Handful parsley   *Bunch up parsley and push*
4 carrots, greens removed   *through hopper with carrots,*
1 garlic clove   *garlic, and celery.*
2 stalks celery

Calcium-Rich Cocktail

3 kale leaves   *Bunch up kale and parsley,*
Small handful parsley   *and push through hopper*
4–5 carrots, greens removed   *with carrots and apple.*
½ apple, seeded

Ginger Hopper

¼-inch slice ginger root   *Push ginger through hopper*
4–5 carrots, greens removed   *with carrots and apple.*
½ apple, seeded

TINNITUS

Tinnitus is a condition in which tinkling or ringing sounds are heard in one or both ears. Individuals who are bothered by these unidentified sounds are often tuning into the mechanics of their own heads. For instance, temperomandibular joint syndrome (TMJ)—an abnormal condition involving facial pain and poor function of the lower jaw—can cause a sound when the jaws move. Other possible causes of perceived noises include impaired movement of blood, inflamed tissues, exposure to environmental toxins, and the use of some drugs. Treatment consists of correcting the underlying physiologic or mechanical problems, eliminating nutrient deficiencies, and removing the offending toxins.

General Recommendations

A variety of drugs, most noticeably aspirin, can cause tinnitus. Check with your pharmacist and physician about any medications you are taking, and discuss the possibility of substituting a different drug. Pollution from your work area may be the problem,and changing to a cleaner, less toxic environment may be the solution. If you think that TMJ might be the problem, ask your dentist for an evaluation. If you suspect that inflamed tissues might be to blame, see your doctor. (*See also* INFLAMMATION in Part Two.)

Dietary Modifications

1. Start your nutritional program with a cleansing diet to detoxify your body. (See page 299.)

2. After completing the cleansing diet, follow the Basic Diet. (See page 285.) Reducing fat and cholesterol through this diet may increase blood flow and better nourish the ear area.

3. Eat fatty fish, such as mackerel and salmon, three or four times a week. The omega-3 fatty acids in these fish improve blood flow in the inner ear.

4. Correct any existing anemias. Iron deficiency and pernicious anemias can cause noises from the jugular vein. (*See* ANEMIA in Part Two.)

5. Limit the amount of simple sugars consumed, including those found in fruit juices. Hypoglycemia, a condition that is worsened by the consumption of sugar, can cause ear ringing and hearing loss. (*See* HYPOGLYCEMIA in Part Two for information on hypoglycemia management.)

Nutrients That Help

☐ **Iron, vitamin B$_{12}$, and folic acid** correct anemias. B$_{12}$ must be taken as a supplement, since no fruit or vegetable provides this nutrient.

☐ **Chromium** helps to correct hypoglycemia by regulating glucose metabolism. Brewer's yeast is an excellent source of this nutrient.

☐ **Manganese** deficiency has been linked with tinnitus.

☐ **Choline** deficiency has been linked with tinnitus.

Beneficial Juices

☐ Beet—a potent detoxifier.

☐ Kale and parsley—sources of iron.

☐ Spinach, kale, beet greens, and sweet pepper—sources of folic acid.

☐ Green pepper and apple—sources of chromium

☐ Spinach, turnip greens, and beet greens—sources of manganese.

☐ Green bean—source of choline.

Suggested Juicing Recipes / Tinnitus

Apple Shake

½ orange, peeled (leave white pithy part)
2 green apples, seeded
1 ripe banana
1 Tbsp. brewer's yeast
Orange slice for garnish

Juice orange and apple. Place juice, banana, and yeast in blender or food processor, and blend until smooth. Garnish with orange slice.

Body Cleanser

½ cucumber
1 beet
½ apple, seeded
4 carrots, greens removed

Push cucumber, beet, and apple through hopper with carrots.

Cherie's Cleansing Cocktail

¼-inch slice ginger root
1 beet
½ apple, seeded
4 carrots, greens removed

Push ginger, beet, and apple through hopper with carrots.

Mineral Tonic

Handful parsley
2 turnip leaves
1 kale leaf
4–5 carrots, greens removed

Roll up parsley in turnip and kale leaves, and push through hopper with carrots.

Three-Bean Juice

Small handful mung and
   lentil sprouts
2 carrots, greens removed
½ cup green beans
1 tomato
Carrot curls for garnish

Bunch up sprouts and push through hopper with carrots, beans, and tomatoes. Garnish with carrot curls.

Waldorf Salad

1 green apple, seeded
1 stalk celery

Push apple and celery through hopper.

ULCERATIVE COLITIS

See COLITIS.

ULCERS

A peptic ulcer is an erosion produced by stomach secretions containing pepsin, an enzyme that speeds the breakdown of protein, and gastric juice, which is mainly composed of hydrochloric acid. Ulcers are usually found in the lining of the stomach or in the first part of the duodenum. The stomach is normally able to protect itself from its own secretions, but when an area of the lining is injured, the acids and enzymes digest the tissue as they would any piece of meat, causing a depression or hole in the stomach or duodenal wall. This injury can be the result of an infection caused by the bacteria *Helicobacter pylori,* or it may result from the ingestion of certain substances such as alcohol and various nonsteroidal anti–inflammatory drugs, including aspirin, Motrin, and Indocin. Remember that while juice therapy helps heal individual ulcers, it will not "cure" a person of ulcer disease. Only identifying and eliminating the cause of the ulcer will result in a permanent cure.

General Recommendations

Contrary to popular belief, stress does not cause ulcers. It can, however, aggravate the condition. If you are the kind of person who takes out life's frustrations on your stomach, stress-reduction techniques may make you feel much more comfortable and may also heal existing ulcers more quickly. If your doctor recommends antacids, be sure to follow package directions. Used incorrectly, these drugs can cause kidney stones and a variety of other problems.

Dietary Modifications

1. Follow the Basic Diet (see page 285), eliminating any foods that cause discomfort. Formerly, ulcer patients were automatically put on a bland diet that was high in milk. Today we know that a bland diet has no effect on ulcer healing or discomfort, and that milk actually makes ulcers worse.

2. Eat a high-fiber diet. Substitute whole grains for refined flour products, and eat a variety of fresh fruits and vegetables. This may help prevent a recurrence of ulcers.

3. Avoid drinking coffee. A recent study has shown that both decaffeinated coffee and regular coffee can cause ulcer-like symptoms.

4. If you must take nonsteroidal anti–inflammatory drugs—for arthritis or for another type of inflammation—make ginger drinks a regular part of each day. Ginger root may help protect the stomach lining from the damage that is sometimes caused by these drugs.

5. Drink cabbage juice, the most famous natural remedy for ulcers. Some people find this juice very soothing, and some find that it stings. If you experience discomfort, start with a cup a day and work up to the recommended quart. Green cabbage works better than red and is much milder in flavor.

According to Dr. Garnett Cheney, only fresh green cabbage heads should be chosen for juicing. Long periods of transportation, particularly in the absence of refrigeration, may lead to destruction of the healing factor. One quart of juice should be drunk each day until the ulcer heals. The juice should be taken in four or five individual servings of six or eight ounces each. Ideally, it should be served five times daily: in the middle of the morning with crackers, with lunch, in the middle of the afternoon with crackers, with the evening meal, and at about eight or nine o'clock with crackers. The juice should not be taken on an empty stomach.

The raw cabbage juice may be made more palatable for some individuals by the addition of celery juice, which also contains the healing factor. Pineapple juice is also a good flavoring agent.

Cabbage juice should never be heated, as this destroys the healing factor. However, frozen cabbage juice held at 32°F (0°C) maintains its antipeptic-ulcer activity for at least three weeks.

The juice may be prepared once or twice each day and stored in the refrigerator. It should not be held overnight because of the strong flavors and odors that develop after standing even a few hours. Cabbage juice is at its best when it is prepared fresh just before drinking. (See the recipe for Dr. Cheney's Ulcer Drink on page 269.)

6. *Check for food sensitivities.* Some studies suggest that chronic ulcers may be due to an allergic response. Try the Elimination Diet, found on page 296.

7. *Eat more bananas.* Some animal studies have shown that bananas can protect the stomach lining from acid.

8. *Add whole-milk yogurt to your diet.* Whole-milk yogurt has been reported to protect the stomach against irritants such as cigarette smoke and alcohol.

Nutrients That Help

☐ **Beta-carotene** is a healing nutrient.

☐ **Vitamin E** is a healing nutrient. Speak to your doctor about supplementation in therapeutic amounts.

☐ **Zinc** is a healing nutrient. Speak to your doctor about supplementation in therapeutic amounts.

☐ **Vitamin C** deficiency is associated with stomach ulcers.

Beneficial Juices

☐ Cantaloupe, spinach, and carrot—sources of beta-carotene.

☐ Kale, red pepper, and collard greens—sources of vitamin C.

☐ Cabbage and celery—sources of the ulcer-healing factor.

☐ Ginger root—may protect stomach lining from drug injury.

Suggested Juicing Recipes / Ulcers

Dr. Cheney's Ulcer Drink

½ head green cabbage
1 stalk celery
½ apple, seeded

Juice vegetables and apple. Drink 2–3 times a day until ulcer is healed.

Monkey Shake

½ orange, peeled (leave white pithy part)
½ papaya, peeled
1 banana
Orange twist for garnish

Push orange through hopper with papaya. Place juice and banana in blender or food processor, and blend until smooth. Garnish with orange twist.

Spicy Cantaloupe Shake

¼-inch slice ginger root
½ cantaloupe, with skin

Push ginger through hopper with cantaloupe.

Ginger Tea

2-inch slice ginger root
¼ lemon
1 pint water
1 stick cinnamon, broken
4–5 cloves
Dash nutmeg or cardamom

Juice ginger and lemon. Place juice in saucepan, and add water, cinnamon, and cloves. Gently simmer. Add nutmeg or cardamom.

Healing Smoothie

1 firm kiwi, peeled
¼ cantaloupe, with skin
1 ripe banana

Push kiwi and cantaloupe through hopper. Place juice and banana in blender or food processor, and blend until smooth. This drink protects and heals the stomach lining.

Mineral Tonic

Handful parsley
2 turnip leaves
1 kale leaf
4–5 carrots, greens removed

*Roll up parsley in turnip and
kale leaves, and push
through hopper with carrots.*

Sweet and Sour Cherry Cream

1 cup cherries, pitted
4 oz. nonfat yogurt

*Juice cherries. Place juice and
yogurt in blender or food
processor, and blend until
smooth.*

UNDERWEIGHT

Successful weight gain depends upon the cause of the initial
weight loss. Some people are genetically programmed to be
thin, and weight gain for them is very difficult. Statistically
speaking, underweight people live longer and have fewer
health problems than overweight individuals. In older adults,
however, thinness can be a reflection of undernourishment.

General Recommendations

Sudden weight loss should always be evaluated by your
physician. Weight loss due to cancer needs special consideration. (*See* CANCER in Part Two.) Weight loss due to lack of
appetite is common in people on drug therapies. Check with
your doctor or pharmacist if you suspect that this is the
problem. Exercise is the best way for the naturally thin person
to shape up. "Recreational" drugs and alcohol can cause
weight loss, and abstinence is the only solution in this instance. If you smoke, stop. Nicotine increases the metabolic
rate.

Dietary Modifications

1. *Follow the Basic Diet.* (See page 285.)

2. *Increase calories by adding complex carbohydrates such as whole grain pasta, potatoes, and bananas to your diet.* Don't add high amounts of fats, as this will only increase your risk of developing cancer or heart disease.

3. *Drink your calories instead of eating them.* Try the high-calorie body builders on the next page. Often it's easier to drink more food than it is to eat it.

4. *Eliminate caffeine-containing beverages, such as coffee, tea, and some colas.* These beverages increase the metabolic rate.

Nutrients That Help

☐ **Zinc** deficiency causes a loss of taste that may contribute to loss of appetite.

Beneficial Juices

☐ Ginger, parsley, and carrot—sources of zinc.

☐ Lemon—a traditional appetite stimulant.

☐ Carrot, kale, and parsley—mineral-rich juices that provide the nutrients the body needs to nourish itself.

☐ Cantaloupe, pineapple, and grape—natural sources of sugar, which boosts calorie levels.

Suggested Juicing Recipes / Underweight

Lemon Spritzer

1 small lemon
Sparkling water

Push lemon through hopper. Pour juice into ice-filled glass. Fill glass to top with sparkling water.

Strawberry Shake

1 pint strawberries
½ firm pear
1 ripe banana
1 Tbsp. brewer's yeast

Push strawberries and pear through hopper. Place juice, banana, and yeast in blender or food processor, and blend until smooth.

Sweet and Sour Cherry Cream

1 cup cherries, pitted
4 oz. nonfat yogurt

Juice cherries. Place juice and yogurt in blender or food processor, and blend until smooth.

Tropical Nectar

1 passion fruit, peeled
½ papaya, peeled
1 nectarine
1 banana
Orange slice for garnish

Push passion fruit, papaya, and nectarine through hopper. Place juice, banana, and ice in blender or food processor, and blend into frosty drink. Garnish with orange slice.

Mineral Tonic

Handful parsley
2 turnip leaves
1 kale leaf
4–5 carrots, greens removed

Roll up parsley in turnip and kale leaves, and push through hopper with carrots.

Red Crush

1 medium bunch red grapes
½ cup cherries, pitted
½ cup blueberries
Handful whole berries (any kind)

Juice grapes, cherries, and berries. Pour juice into a glass or bowl over finely crushed ice. Sprinkle whole berries on top, and eat with a spoon.

Blueberry Shake

1 pint blueberries
1 ripe banana
2 Tbsp. protein powder

Juice blueberries. Place juice, banana, and protein powder in blender or food processor, and blend until smooth.

Ginger Hopper

¼-inch slice ginger root
4–5 carrots, greens removed
½ apple, seeded

Push ginger through hopper with carrots and apple.

URINARY TRACT INFECTION

See BLADDER INFECTION.

VAGINITIS

See CANDIDIASIS.

VARICOSE VEINS

Varicose veins are veins that are widened, distended, and, in some cases, twisted. Usually, this condition is the result of a breakdown of the valves inside the veins. When the valves no longer work properly, blood stagnates and accumulates in the veins, stretching them and causing varicosity. The most common site for this disorder is the superficial veins of the legs, just under the skin. Because the superficial veins are so easily injured, these veins may bleed into the surrounding tissues, causing blood clots, swelling, and the formation of ulcers on the lower part of the leg. More common symptoms include dull, nagging aches and pains and a feeling of heaviness in the legs.

Hemorrhoids are varicose veins of the anus or rectum. Symptoms of this disorder include rectal itching and pain, and blood in the stools. Hemorrhoids are usually caused by constipation and improper diet.

General Recommendations

To reduce the pressure on the valves in the veins of the legs, avoid standing in one place too long. If your occupation puts a lot of stress on your legs or if you are pregnant, wear support stockings. Exercise on a regular basis, and reduce weight if necessary. If you suffer from hemorrhoids, dietary changes may be your best weapon.

Dietary Modifications

1. Follow the Basic Diet. (See page 285.)

2. Consume a diet that is high in fiber. A high-fiber diet is thought to be helpful because it decreases the need to strain when having bowel movements.

3. Eat more ginger, garlic, and onions. These foods help to break down the fibrin surrounding the varicose vein. People with varicose veins have a decreased ability to break down this substance.

Nutrients That Help

☐ **Bromelain** aids in activating a factor that promotes the breakdown of fibrin. Bromelain also prevents the formation of blood clots.

☐ **Anthocyanins and proanthocyanidins** are pigments found in dark-colored berries. These substances may help to strengthen the venous wall and increase the muscular tone of the vein.

☐ **Beta-carotene** is a healing nutrient.

☐ **Vitamin E** is a healing nutrient. Speak to your doctor about supplementation in therapeutic amounts.

☐ **Zinc** is a healing nutrient. Speak to your doctor about supplementation in therapeutic amounts.

Beneficial Juices

☐ Pineapple—a source of bromelain.

☐ Cherry, blueberry, and blackberry—sources of anthocyanins and proanthocyanidins.

☐ Kale, parsley, and collard greens—great sources of beta-carotene.

☐ Garlic and onion—sources of an anticlotting factor.

☐ Ginger—has anti-inflammatory and anticlotting properties.

☐ Cantaloupe—a source of beta-carotene and of an anticlotting factor.

Suggested Juicing Recipes / Varicose Veins

Garlic Express

Handful parsley
1 garlic clove
4–5 carrots, greens removed
2 stalks celery

Bunch up parsley and push through hopper with garlic, carrots, and celery.

Cherry Smile

1 cup cherries, pitted
¼ lime
1 medium bunch green
    grapes
Lime twist for garnish

Juice cherries, lime, and grapes. Pour juice into tall glass over crushed ice, and garnish with lime twist.

Cantaloupe Shake

½ cantaloupe, with skin

Cut cantaloupe in strips, and push through hopper.

High-Calcium Drink

3 kale leaves
Small handful parsley
4–5 carrots, greens removed

Bunch up kale and parsley, and push through hopper with carrots.

Maureen's Spicy Tonic

¼ pineapple, with skin
½ apple, seeded
¼-inch slice ginger root

Push pineapple through hopper with apple and ginger.

Healing Smoothie

1 firm kiwi, peeled
¼ cantaloupe, with skin
1 ripe banana

Push kiwi and cantaloupe through hopper. Place juice and banana in blender or food processor, and blend until smooth. This drink protects and heals the stomach lining.

Tossed Salad

1 kale leaf
1 turnip leaf
Handful spinach
2 tomatoes
1 cherry tomato for garnish

Bunch up the leaves and spinach, and push through hopper with tomatoes. Garnish with cherry tomato.

WATER RETENTION

Most women and older men have suffered at one time or another from water retention, or edema. Edema is the pooling of water in the tissues. Although it often occurs in the hands and feet, any part of the body may have edema. This retention of water has a number of possible causes, including birth control pills, premenstrual syndrome, pregnancy, kidney disease, and food allergies. Natural diuretics gently promote the loss of water, reducing the swelling.

Caution: Care must be taken to apply these remedies only to mild cases of edema. Swelling of the ankles in particular can be an indication of heart failure, and must be treated by a physician immediately. If you have any questions about the seriousness of your condition, contact your doctor. If your doctor prescribes diuretics, check with your doctor or pharmacist to see if the medication you're taking is potassium-sparing. Individuals who take potassium-sparing diuretics should avoid potassium supplements and high-potassium foods. Individuals who take diuretics that are not potassium-sparing need to consume high-potassium foods.

Dietary Modifications

1. Follow the Basic Diet. (See page 285.)

2. Decrease the amount of salt in your diet. This can be easily done by eliminating the use of table salt as a seasoning and avoiding convenience foods and snack foods. When cooking, use lemon to add zest without adding salt. Do not buy snacks that are marked "low salt" or "light salt." Buy snacks that are whole grain and contain *no* added salt, including sea salt. Pregnant women should *not* reduce the amount of salt in their diet. Low-sodium diets are associated with complications of pregnancy.

3. Decrease or eliminate white sugar. Animal studies have implicated sucrose in cases of excess sodium retention.

4. Consider the possibility that you have an allergy. Water retention, particularly around the eyes, can be a sign of food intolerance. (*See* ALLERGIES in Part Two.)

5. Eat generous portions of foods traditionally used as diuretics: artichokes, cantaloupe, watermelon, garlic, and dill.

Nutrients That Help

☐ **Potassium** should be increased through the consumption of potassium-rich foods if you are on diuretics that do not spare potassium. This mineral also helps counteract the effects of sodium in water retention. Individuals taking diuretics that do spare potassium should avoid potassium-rich foods and potassium supplements.

☐ **Magnesium** is lost as a result of diuretic pills and must be replaced.

☐ **Vitamin B₆** deficiency may limit the kidneys' ability to secrete sodium.

Beneficial Juices

☐ Parsley, Swiss chard, spinach, broccoli, kale, carrot, and celery—good sources of potassium.

☐ Collard, parsley, and garlic—sources of magnesium.

☐ Kale, spinach, turnip greens, and sweet pepper—sources of vitamin B₆.

☐ Watermelon, cucumber, grape, lettuce, and cantaloupe (with seeds)—traditional, gentle diuretics.

☐ Garlic—a traditional remedy for water retention.

Suggested Juicing Recipes / Water Retention

Cucumber Cooler

1 tomato	*Juice tomato, pour juice into*
1 cucumber	*ice cube tray, and freeze.*
2 stalks celery	*Juice cucumber and celery.*
Parsley sprig for garnish	*Pour juice into tall glass, add*
	tomato cubes, and garnish
	with sprig of parsley.

Summer Breeze

1 orange, peeled (leave white
  pithy part)
1 medium bunch green
  grapes
2 cups watermelon pieces,
  with rind
Mint sprig for garnish

*Push orange, grapes, and
watermelon through hopper.
Pour juice into tall glass over
crushed ice, and garnish with
sprig of mint.*

Folk Remedy Diuretic

2 large apples, seeded
½ tsp. horseradish

*Juice apples and mix with
horseradish. Drink three
times a day.*

Sweet Potassium Shake

¼ cantaloupe
1 banana

*Juice cantaloupe. Place juice
and banana in blender or
food processor, and blend
until smooth.*

Potassium Broth

Handful parsley
Handful spinach
4–5 carrots, greens removed
2 stalks celery

*Bunch up parsley and
spinach leaves, and push
through hopper with carrots
and celery.*

Garden Salad Special

3 broccoli flowerets
1 garlic clove
4–5 carrots or 2 tomatoes
2 stalks celery
½ green pepper

*Push broccoli and garlic
through hopper with carrots
or tomatoes. Follow with
celery and green pepper.*

Strawberry Shake

1 pint strawberries
½ firm pear
1 ripe banana
1 Tbsp. brewer's yeast

Push strawberries and pear through hopper. Place juice, banana, and yeast in blender or food processor, and blend until smooth.

Body Cleanser

½ cucumber
1 beet
½ apple, seeded
4 carrots, greens removed

Push cucumber, beet, and apple through hopper with carrots.

WEIGHT PROBLEMS

See OVERWEIGHT/OBESITY; UNDERWEIGHT.

WOUND HEALING

See SURGERY PREPARATION.

YEAST INFECTIONS

See CANDIDIASIS.

PART THREE

The Diet Plans

Introduction

When you are sick, the food you eat is never neutral. It
can either contribute to or hinder your recovery. Similarly, when you are well, your diet can help your body remain
strong, or it can leave you susceptible to infection or other
disorders. Several of the diets in this section are suitable for
daily use. Fine-tune them by adding the juices recommended
in the appropriate sections of Part Two, and you'll have a
personalized program that will support you when you're ill and
help you maintain your health. A few diets, such as the Juice
Fast (see page 301) and the Elimination Diet (see page 296),
are designed for short-term use only. These diets can be used
to cleanse your body of toxins, to identify food allergies, to help
you lose unwanted weight, and to boost your immune system
in times of illness.

Remember that these diets are intended to supplement your
physician's recommendations, and should never be used in
lieu of medical care. Always consult your physician before
beginning a new nutritional program.

Diets for Everyday Use

THE BASIC DIET

This diet is designed for everyday use, both in times of illness and in times of good health. By referring to the recommendations in Part Two, you will be able to tailor the diet to meet your needs. Simply write the recommended juices from Part Two in the blanks provided in the diet plan. Be aware that the small number of recommended servings is intended for women, the larger number for men. If you find you are losing weight, add more servings or increase serving size.

SUGGESTED MENU

Breakfast

Juice: _____
Hot cereal with skim milk
Piece of fruit
Whole grain toast
Tea

Mid-Morning Snack

Juice: _____
Nut butter on
  whole wheat crackers

Lunch

Juice: _____

Vegetable salad
Bean or pea soup
Sandwich

Mid-Afternoon Snack

Juice: _____

Apple wedges

Dinner

Juice: _____

Green salad
Stir-fry with vegetables and
  meat, poultry, or seafood
Baked potato
Whole grain roll

Evening Snack

Juice: _____

Yogurt

BASIC DIET GUIDELINES

Below you will find a list of the food groups that make up the Basic Diet. For each group—Cereals, Grains, Breads, and Potatoes, for instance—we have specified those foods that are recommended on this diet, and those foods that should be avoided.

☐ **Cereals, Grains, Breads, Potatoes** (2–5 servings per meal)

Recommended Foods: All whole grains, such as whole wheat, millet, rye, cornmeal, buckwheat, brown rice. Wheat germ, bran. Steamed or baked potatoes. Low-fat whole grain chips and crackers. Whole wheat pasta and noodles. Air-popped popcorn.

Foods to Avoid: White breads or crackers, refined or sugared cereals. Fried potatoes, potato chips, corn chips. Buttered popcorn. Cake, cookies, donuts. Refined flour pasta and noodles.

☐ **Beans** (3–5 cups per week. Strict vegetarians should eat 2–3 cups per day.)

Recommended Foods: Legumes (e.g., kidney, pinto, lentils). Sprouts. All soy products (e.g., tofu, soymilk).

Foods to Avoid: Fast-food refried beans with added lard. Check before you order.

☐ Nuts and Seeds (1–2 servings per week)

Recommended Foods: All nuts, seeds, and nut butters.

Foods to Avoid: Peanut butter with added oil and sugar. Nuts roasted in oil or salted.

☐ Vegetables (4–8 servings per day)

A serving of vegetables equals ½ cup whole produce or 6 ounces juice. A minimum of 8 glasses of fluids should be consumed every day.

Recommended Foods: All fresh raw or lightly steamed vegetables. Fresh vegetable juices.

Foods to Avoid: Canned vegetables. Canned or bottled vegetable juices. Fried vegetables.

☐ Fruit (3–5 servings or pieces per day)

A serving of fruit equals ½ cup whole produce or 6 ounces juice. A minimum of 8 glasses of fluids should be consumed every day.

Recommended Foods: All fresh raw or cooked fruits eaten whole. All fresh fruit juices.

Foods to Avoid: Canned, sweetened fruits. Canned, bottled, or frozen juices.

☐ Milk Products (as desired)

Recommended Foods: Low-fat dairy products, skim milk, non-fat yogurt.

Foods to Avoid: Whole milk, sweetened yogurt, ice cream, sour cream.

☐ Meat (3 oz. per day no more than once or twice a week), Poultry (3–4 oz. per day), or Seafood (6 oz. per day)

Recommended Foods: Lean meats. Skinless poultry (white meat). All fish and shellfish.

Foods to Avoid: Lunch or canned meats, hot dogs, bacon, sausage, organ meats. Charbroiled meats. Fried chicken. Poultry skin. All deep-fried seafood.

☐ **Cheese** (no more than 1–2 oz. per day)

Recommended Foods: Low- or nonfat cheese, low-fat cottage cheese.

Foods to Avoid: All whole-milk cheese, whole cottage cheese.

☐ **Fats** (4–7 tsp. per day)

Recommended Foods: Cold-pressed canola oil, high-oleic safflower oil, olive oil, flaxseed oil. Dressings and mayonnaise made with the above oils.

Foods to Avoid: Margarine, shortening, tropical oils. All animal fats. Nondairy creamers.

☐ **Miscellaneous**

Recommended Foods: Herbal teas, water, green or black teas (decaffeinated). Garlic, ginger, pepper. All soy products such as soymilk, tofu, tempeh, low-salt soy sauce. Low-sugar jams and jellies in small amounts.

Foods to Avoid: Coffee, soft drinks, fruit drinks, sweets, salt.

THE SUGAR METABOLISM DISORDER DIET

This variation of the Basic Diet is low in simple sugars and high in complex carbohydrates. Eating in this manner will help to slow the release of sugar into the blood stream, keeping blood glucose levels more even and blood fats lowered. This is extremely important for diabetics and hypoglycemics. On this diet, you should never drink fruit juices full strength or on an empty stomach, as this can cause a sudden rise in blood sugar levels.

Caution: If you are a diabetic on insulin, you must check with your doctor before making any changes in your diet. This menu is intended only as a guide and is not meant to replace the diet prescribed by your doctor.

SUGGESTED MENU

Breakfast

Juice: _____
High-fiber cold cereal with
  skim milk
Whole grain toast with 2 tsp.
  Better Butter (see page 62)
Herbal tea

Mid-Morning Snack

Juice: _____
Whole wheat crackers

Lunch

Juice: _____
Whole wheat pita bread with
  hummus spread and sprouts
Green salad with tomatoes
  and 1 Tbsp. dressing

Mid-Afternoon Snack

Juice: _____
Low-fat yogurt

Dinner

Juice: _____
Pasta with clam sauce
Steamed vegetables
Whole grain roll with 1 tsp.
  Better Butter
Garden salad with nonfat
  dressing

Evening Snack

Juice: _____
3 cups air-popped popcorn

SUGAR METABOLISM DISORDER DIET GUIDELINES

Below you will find a list of the food groups that make up the Sugar Metabolism Disorder Diet. For each group—Cereals, Grains, Breads, and Potatoes, for instance—we have specified those foods that are recommended on this diet, and those foods that should be avoided.

☐ **Cereals, Grains, Breads, Potatoes** (3–6 servings per meal)

Recommended Foods: All whole grains, such as whole wheat, millet, rye, cornmeal, buckwheat, brown rice. Wheat germ, bran. Steamed or baked potatoes. Low-fat whole grain chips and crackers. Whole wheat pasta and noodles. Air-popped popcorn.

Foods to Avoid: White breads or crackers, refined or sugared cereals. Fried potatoes, potato chips, corn chips. Buttered popcorn. Cake, cookies, or donuts. Refined flour pasta and noodles.

☐ **Beans** (5–7 cups per week. Strict vegetarians should eat 2–3 cups per day.)

Recommended Foods: Legumes (e.g., kidney, pinto, lentils). Sprouts. All soy products (e.g., tofu, soymilk, tempeh).

Foods to Avoid: Fast-food refried beans with added lard. Check before you order.

☐ **Nuts and Seeds** (1–2 servings per week)

Recommended Foods: All nuts, seeds, and nut butters.

Foods to Avoid: Peanut butter with added oil and sugar. Nuts roasted in oil or salted.

☐ **Vegetables** (5–9 servings per day)

A serving of vegetables equals ½ cup whole produce or 6 ounces juice. A minimum of 8 glasses of fluids should be consumed each day.

Recommended Foods: All fresh raw or lightly steamed vegetables. Fresh vegetable juices. Drink carrot juice with meals only.

Foods to Avoid: Canned vegetables. Canned or bottled vegetable juices. Fried vegetables.

☐ **Fruit** (1–3 servings or pieces per week)

A serving of fruit equals ½ cup whole produce or 6 ounces juice. A minimum of 8 glasses of fluids should be consumed each day.

Recommended Foods: All fresh raw or cooked fruits eaten whole. All fresh fruit juices when diluted with water and drunk with meals.

Foods to Avoid: Canned, sweetened fruits. Canned, bottled, or frozen juices. Sherbet, jam, jelly, honey, white sugar. All concentrated sources of sugar.

☐ **Milk Products** (as desired)

Recommended Foods: Low-fat dairy products, skim milk, non-fat yogurt.

Foods to Avoid: Whole milk, sweetened yogurt, ice cream, sour cream.

☐ **Meat** (3 oz. per day no more than once or twice a week), **Poultry** (3–4 oz. per day), **or Seafood** (6 oz. per day)

Recommended Foods: Lean meats. Skinless poultry (white meat). All fish and shellfish.

Foods to Avoid: Lunch or canned meats, hot dogs, organ meats, bacon, sausage. Charbroiled meats. Fried chicken. Poultry skin. All deep-fried seafood.

☐ **Cheese** (no more than 1–2 oz. per day)

Recommended Foods: Low- or nonfat cheese, low-fat cottage cheese.

Foods to Avoid: All whole-milk cheese, whole cottage cheese.

☐ **Fats** (4–7 tsp. per day)

Recommended Foods: Cold-pressed canola oil, high-oleic safflower oil, flaxseed oil. Dressings and mayonnaise made with the above oils.

Foods to Avoid: Margarine, shortening, tropical oils. All animal fats.

☐ **Miscellaneous**

Recommended Foods: Herbal teas, water, black or green teas (decaffeinated). Garlic, ginger, pepper. All soy products including soymilk, tofu, tempeh.

Foods to Avoid: Coffee, soft drinks, fruit drinks, sweets.

Special Needs Diets

THE IMMUNE SUPPORT DIET

The immune support diet is intended for the times that your body's immune system is under attack. If you find yourself unable to eat solid foods, add one of the high-protein drinks to replace the protein lost during your illness. A minimum of eight glasses of fluids should be drunk during the day as water, juice, or broth. Sugar of any kind may depress the immune system, so eliminate all sweets.

SUGGESTED MENU

Breakfast

Juice: _____
Raw or cooked unsweetened
  fruit, 1/2 serving
Whole grain hot or cold cereal
  with nonfat milk
Whole grain toast
Green tea

Mid-Morning Snack

Juice: _____
Whole grain low-fat crackers

Lunch

Juice: _____

Salad of leafy greens with
  garlic dressing
Broth or soup
Sandwich
Herbal tea

Mid-Afternoon Snack

Juice: _____

Yogurt

Dinner

Juice: _____

Broiled or baked cold-water
  fish
Steamed vegetables
Brown rice

Evening Snack

Juice: _____

IMMUNE SUPPORT DIET GUIDELINES

Below you will find a list of the food groups that make up the
Immune Support Diet. For each group—Cereals, Grains, Breads,
and Potatoes, for instance—we have specified those foods that
are recommended on this diet, and those foods that should be
avoided.

☐ **Cereals, Grains, Breads, Potatoes** (2–5 servings per meal)

Recommended Foods: All whole grains, such as whole wheat,
millet, rye, cornmeal, buckwheat, brown rice. Wheat germ,
bran. Steamed or baked potatoes. Low-fat whole grain chips
and crackers. Whole wheat pasta and noodles. Air-popped
popcorn.

Foods to Avoid: White breads or crackers, refined or sugared
cereals. Fried potatoes, potato chips, corn chips. Buttered
popcorn. Cakes, cookies, donuts. Refined flour pasta and
noodles.

☐ **Beans** (3–5 cups per week. Strict vegetarians should eat
2–3 cups per day.)

Recommended Foods: Legumes (e.g., kidney, pinto, lentils).
Sprouts. All soy products (e.g., tofu, soymilk).

Foods to Avoid: Fast-food refried beans with added lard. Check before you order.

☐ **Nuts and Seeds** (1–2 servings per day)

Recommended Foods: All nuts, seeds, and nut butters.

Foods to Avoid: Peanut butter with added oil and sugar.

☐ **Vegetables** (4–8 servings per day)
A serving of vegetables equals 1/2 cup whole produce or 6 ounces juice. A minimum of 8 glasses of fluids should be consumed every day.

Recommended Foods: All fresh raw or lightly steamed vegetables and juices, with emphasis on cabbage, kale, carrot, pepper, collard, garlic.

Foods to Avoid: Canned vegetables. Canned or bottled vegetable juices. Fried vegetables.

☐ **Fruit** (2–4 servings or pieces per week)
A serving of fruit equals 1/2 cup whole produce or 6 ounces juice. A minimum of 8 glasses of fluids should be consumed every day.

Recommended Foods: All fresh fruits or juices, with emphasis on apple, pineapple, blueberry, grape.

Foods to Avoid: Canned, sweetened fruits. Canned, bottled, or frozen juices.

☐ **Milk Products** (as desired)

Recommended Foods: Low-fat dairy products, skim milk, non-fat yogurt.

Foods to Avoid: Whole milk, sweetened yogurt, ice cream, sour cream.

☐ **Meat** (None), **Poultry** (3–4 oz. per day), **or Seafood** (6 oz. per day)

Recommended Foods: Skinless poultry. All fish and shellfish. Emphasize cold-water fatty fish such as mackerel and salmon.

Foods to Avoid: All beef, veal, pork, lunch meats, hot dogs, organ meats. Fried chicken. Poultry skin. All deep-fried seafood.

☐ **Cheese** (no more than 1–2 oz. per day)

Recommended Foods: Low- or nonfat cheese, low-fat cottage cheese.

Foods to Avoid: All whole-milk cheese, whole cottage cheese.

☐ **Fats** (4–7 tsp. per day)

Recommended Foods: Cold-pressed canola oil, high-oleic safflower oil, olive oil, flaxseed oil. Dressings and mayonnaise made with the above oils.

Foods to Avoid: Margarine, shortening, tropical oils. All animal fats. Nondairy creamers.

☐ **Miscellaneous**

Recommended Foods: Herbal teas, water. Garlic, ginger, pepper. Black or green tea if limited to one cup per day.

Foods to Avoid: Coffee, soft drinks, fruit drinks, sweets.

THE ELIMINATION DIET

This diet is designed to help you identify food allergies and sensitivities. For the first seven days (the cleansing period), eat only the foods listed in the following plan. Symptoms due to food allergies should disappear during this time. If not, factors other than food may be involved, or some unapproved food may have been eaten. Another possibility is that you have an allergy to one of the approved foods. This occurs in only a very small number of people, but it does happen. Lamb, rye, peaches, sweet potatoes, or tea is usually at fault. Restrictions of the foods in this diet should be attempted only under a doctor's supervision, however.

If progress is noticed during the week, it is advisable to continue on this diet another two or three days. During this period, avoid all other foods. Read labels on all products to make sure that no forbidden foods or additives have been used. The following foods may be eaten in the desired amount, so you don't have to worry about being hungry. At the end of the diet period, symptoms are usually gone, and you can begin to reintroduce other foods, one at a time. Make a note of any symptoms that follow the ingestion of a food, and avoid those foods that cause problems. And remember that some reactions can be delayed.

SUGGESTED MENU

Breakfast
Apricot or prune juice
Stewed prunes
Brown rice cereal with juice
   substituted for milk

Rice bread, toasted
Willow Run margarine
Herbal tea

Lunch

Baked sweet potato
Beets or beet greens
Broiled lamb chop
Rice cakes

Ripe olives
Peaches
Herbal tea

Dinner

Spinach
Brown rice
Spinach salad with only ap-
   proved condiments

Roast lamb
Apricots
Herbal tea

ELIMINATION DIET GUIDELINES

☐ **Allowed Condiments**. Sea salt and white vinegar.

☐ **Allowed Beverages**. Herbal teas.

☐ **Allowed Cereals and Grains**. Rice cereals made with brown rice, such as cream of brown rice. Bread made with rice flour. Rice cakes or plain Ry–Krisp crackers may be used instead of bread.

☐ **Allowed Fruits**. Apricots, peaches, cranberries, prunes (cooked only), cherries (cooked, dry or fresh), and ripe black olives.

☐ **Allowed Fruit Juices**. Apricot, prune, and cranberry—all homemade in your juicer.

☐ **Allowed Fats**. Willow Run margarine, cottonseed oil, and olive oil.

☐ **Allowed Meat**. Lamb.

☐ **Allowed Vegetables**. Sweet potatoes (boiled or baked), beets (fresh or home canned), beet greens (fresh), spinach (fresh, frozen, or home canned), and lettuce. Vegetables must be thoroughly cooked and seasoned only with allowed condiments and fats.

Cleansing Diets

Your body is like a house. It needs regular cleaning and, occasionally, a thorough "spring cleansing" to operate at peak performance. If you want to achieve optimal health and optimal energy, a detoxification plan should be part of your lifestyle. Over time, the body builds up toxins from pesticides and other chemicals, pollution, overindulgences, and body waste. Organs like your liver, kidneys, and colon need continual support. For example, the liver stores some poisons that cannot be broken down and excreted. High amounts of DDT have been found in some people's livers. Signs of toxic buildup include headache, fatigue, depression, belching, flatulence, irritability, insomnia, nausea, abdominal discomfort, tender abdomen, loss of memory or concentration, lack of sexual desire, skin blemishes, sallow complexion, bad breath, coated tongue, body odor, lower back pain, menstrual problems, and aches and pains.

All of the diets presented in this section will cleanse your body safely and effectively. Used faithfully, and in conjunction with enemas and dry brushing when desired, they will help heal your body and allow you to derive the greatest possible benefits from your new juicing program.

ENEMAS

Enemas are very helpful during all cleansing diets. Often, the bowel, kidneys, lungs, and skin are not able to eliminate toxic products fast enough during these diets, and skin eruptions or other symptoms can result. Enemas assist the body in the elimination process and help minimize such symptoms. Although most people today are unfamiliar with enemas, their therapeutic benefits have been known for centuries, and were recorded as early as 1500 B.C. in an ancient Egyptian medical document. Later, in Greece, Hippocrates, the father of medicine, espoused the benefits of enemas. And in this country, in the early part of this century, enemas were commonly used to reverse the onset of illness. After World War II, high-tech medicine turned away from this ancient healing practice. But enemas and colonics (colonics must be administered by a trained technician) are making a comeback as a vital part of the regimen of cleansing the body. For more information on enemas and colon care, see *Prescription for Nutritional Healing* by James and Phyllis Balch, *Healing Within* by Stanley Weinberger, *Colon Health* by Norman Walker, and *Tissue Cleansing Through Bowel Management* by Bernard Jensen.

DRY BRUSHING

Dry brushing the body with a natural-bristle bath brush or loofah mitt each day before bathing can be very beneficial during the cleansing process. The skin is an important organ of elimination, and dry brushing can greatly assist in the task of detoxification. Brush in circular motions, always moving toward the heart. If there are patches of eczema, skin eruptions, or any other skin condition, avoid brushing the affected areas. Also avoid brushing the face.

THE JUICE FAST

Juice fasting is a safe and easy way to detoxify the body. Fasting is not harmful. If it were, mankind would not have evolved as a civilization. Fasts have been recorded in ancient history, and have been a part of virtually all religions. For example, in the orthodox Christian church, fasts have been practiced for centuries and are still a way of church life today.

We do not recommend water fasts because they are too hard on the body. Such fasts release too many stored-up toxins without supplying the nutrients needed to detoxify them. These nutrients, especially the antioxidants (beta-carotene, vitamins C and E, and the mineral selenium) supplied in abundance in the juices, bind with harmful toxins and carry them out of the body.

Some words of caution are in order regarding juice fasting. Children under seventeen should not follow a strict juice fast. But fruit and vegetable juices are a great supplement to a healthful diet for your child or adolescent. Diabetics should seek a doctor's approval before trying a juice fast. The Six-Week Cleansing Diet (see page 313), which is basically a vegan diet, may be appropriate in this case. Hypoglycemics may benefit from using protein powder as a supplement during the fast. Whenever you are sick, your body is sending you a signal that it needs rest—both from strenuous work and from foods that are hard to digest—along with plenty of immune-supporting nutrients. Juices offer great quantities of nutrients that support your immune system, and the juice fast is a powerful healing tool. But don't wait until you are sick to try fasting! We suggest a juice fast several times a year. You can fast from one to five days any time you like. Some people do a two- or three-day cleansing fast every month. If you fast for longer than five days, we suggest you seek qualified supervision.

302 _Juicing for Life_

Drinks that are especially cleansing on the juice fast include beets (no more than three ounces should be consumed the first day, but this amount can be increased gradually up to six ounces), cabbage, wheatgrass, sprouts, lemon, carrot, celery, and apple. In addition, you can add herbal teas such as dandelion root and nettle. These two herbs help cleanse the liver and kidneys. (Steep only 1/2 teaspoon of each herb in a pint of water, strain, and drink warm. Add lemon for flavor.) Vegetable broths can be drunk as well. Gently simmer fresh vegetables with onions and garlic, strain out the vegetables, and add a dash of seasoning to make a nutritious broth you can drink as desired. Also, if you find that you need something to munch on, don't hesitate to modify the fast by adding fresh raw vegetables.

Bulking agents such as psyllium seed husks are used commonly as mucilaginous bulk laxatives. One or two teaspoons can be added to a glass of juice once or twice a day. This can be a very helpful aid to elimination during the cleansing fast.

Breaking the fast properly is as important as the fast itself. If the fast is broken incorrectly, more bad than good can result. Actually, your diet the day before the fast should consist of raw fruits and vegetables with vegetable broths, homemade vegetable soups, or steamed vegetables. No animal products should be consumed until the second day after the fast, when fish as well as whole grains may be added.

The suggested menu, below, is a guideline for the juice fast, which can be followed for one to five consecutive days. This schedule can be modified whenever necessary to meet your individual needs. After the menus, you will find an extensive listing of juice recipes. A Suggested Menu for Breaking the Juice Fast is presented on page 310.

SUGGESTED MENU

Breakfast

Energy Shake, Ginger Hopper, or Pink Morning Tonic

Mid-Morning Snack

Blood Regenerator, Cherie's Cleansing Cocktail, or Green Surprise

Lunch

Zippy Spring Tonic, Year-Round Cleansing Cocktail or Potassium Broth, and Harvest Soup

Mid-Afternoon Snack

Maureen's Spicy Tonic or Digestive Special

Happy Hour

Berry Cantaloupe Shake, Watermelon Juice, or Waldorf Salad

Dinner

Cleansing Tonic, Garden Salad Special, Alkaline Special, and Harvest Soup

Bedtime Snack

Sleepytime tea or chamomile tea

RECIPES FOR JUICE FAST

The following recipes offer possibilities for each "juice meal" of the day. You can choose from one of these recipes or you can make up your own. Feel free to dilute any or all of these juice recipes with water. In fact, many health professionals recommend diluting all fruit juices with an equal amount of water. Finally, we recommend that you have one beet juice and one cabbage juice drink per day because of their effectiveness in cleansing the body. Before trying these or any other juice recipes, read through "Juicing Tips" on page 25.

Breakfast

Energy Shake

Handful parsley
4–6 carrots, greens removed
Parsley sprig for garnish

Bunch up parsley and push through hopper with carrots. Garnish with sprig of parsley.

Ginger Hopper

¼-inch slice ginger root
4–5 carrots, greens removed
½ apple, seeded

*Push ginger through hopper
with carrots and apple.*

Pink Morning Tonic

1 pink grapefruit, peeled
    (leave white pithy part)
1 Red Delicious apple, seeded

*Push grapefruit through
hopper with apple.*

Peach Nectar

2 firm peaches, pitted
1/2 lime
1 ripe banana
1 Tbsp. brewer's yeast

*Juice peaches and lime. Place
juice, banana, and yeast in
blender or food processor,
and blend until smooth.*

Morning Energizer

Handful parsley
5 carrots, greens removed
½ apple, seeded

*Bunch up parsley and push
through hopper with carrots
and apple.*

Mid-Morning Snacks

Green Surprise

1 large kale leaf
2–3 green apples, seeded
Lime twist for garnish

*Bunch up kale leaf and push
through hopper with apples.
Garnish with lime twist. The
surprise is that you won't
taste the kale!*

Cherie's Cleansing Cocktail

¼-inch slice ginger root
1 beet
½ apple, seeded
4 carrots, greens removed

*Push ginger, beet, and apple
through hopper with carrots.*

Blood Regenerator

Handful spinach
4 lettuce leaves
4 sprigs parsley
6 carrots, greens removed
¼ turnip

Bunch up spinach, lettuce, and parsley, and push through hopper with carrots and turnip

Lung Tonic

Small handful parsley
4 sprigs watercress
¼ potato, peeled
6 carrots, greens removed

Bunch up parsley and watercress, and push through hopper with potato and carrots.

Lunch

Zippy Spring Tonic

Handful dandelion greens
   (unsprayed)
3 pineapple rings, with skin
3 radishes

Bunch up dandelion greens and push through hopper with pineapple and radishes.

Potassium Broth

Handful parsley
Handful spinach
4–5 carrots, greens removed
2 stalks celery

Bunch up parsley and spinach leaves, and push through hopper with carrots and celery.

Year-Round Cleansing Cocktail

2 parsley sprigs
Small handful wheatgrass
4–6 carrots, greens removed
2 stalks celery
1 apple, seeded
½ beet

Bunch up parsley and wheatgrass, and push through hopper with carrots, celery, apple, and beet.

Harvest Soup

2–3 garlic cloves
1 kale leaf
1 large tomato
2 stalks celery
1 collard leaf, chopped
1 Tbsp. croutons

Roll garlic in kale leaf, and push through hopper with tomato and celery. Place juice in saucepan, add chopped collards, and gently heat. Garnish with croutons.

Mid-Afternoon Snacks

Maureen's Spicy Tonic

¼ pineapple, with skin
½ apple, seeded
¼-inch slice ginger root

Push pineapple through hopper with apple and ginger.

Digestive Special

Handful spinach
4–5 carrots, greens removed

Bunch up spinach and push through hopper with carrots.

Morning Energizer

Handful parsley
5 carrots, greens removed
½ apple, seeded

Bunch up parsley and push through hopper with carrots and apple.

Liver Mover

1 small beet
2–3 apples, seeded

Push beet and apples through hopper.

Happy Hour

Berry Cantaloupe Shake

½ cantaloupe, with skin
5–6 strawberries

Push cantaloupe and strawberries through hopper.

Watermelon Juice

2-inch slice watermelon, with
  rind
Orange slice for garnish

*Juice watermelon. Pour juice
into glass and garnish with
orange slice.*

Waldorf Salad

1 green apple, seeded
1 stalk celery

*Push apple and celery
through hopper.*

Applemint Fizz

4–6 sprigs fresh mint
2 green apples, seeded
1 small lemon wedge
Sparkling water
Mint sprig for garnish

*Bunch up mint and push
through hopper with apples
and lemon. Juice directly into
a small pitcher filled with ice.
Pour juice into tall glass and
fill with sparkling water.
Garnish with sprig of mint.*

Very Berry Cocktail

1 large bunch grapes
1 quart blueberries or
  blackberries
Sparkling water
Lemon twist for garnish

*Push grapes and berries
through hopper. Juice directly
into small, ice-filled pitcher.
Pour juice into tall glass and
fill glass to top with sparkling
water. Garnish with lemon
twist.*

Dinner

Cleansing Tonic

½-inch wedge green cabbage
2 green apples, seeded
6 carrots, greens removed

*Push cabbage, apples, and
carrots through hopper.*

Alkaline Special

¼ head cabbage (red or
    green)
3 stalks celery

*Push cabbage and celery
through hopper.*

Garden Salad Special

3 broccoli flowerets
1 garlic clove
4–5 carrots or 2 tomatoes
2 stalks celery
½ green pepper

*Push broccoli and garlic
through hopper with carrots
or tomatoes. Follow with
celery and green pepper.*

Maureen's Secret

Handful parsley
2–3 garlic cloves
3 stalks celery
3 carrots, greens removed

*Bunch up parsley and push
through hopper with garlic,
celery, and carrots.*

Harvest Soup

2–3 garlic cloves
1 kale leaf
1 large tomato
2 stalks celery
1 collard leaf, chopped
1 Tbsp. croutons

*Roll garlic in kale leaf, and
push through hopper with
tomato and celery. Place juice
in saucepan, add chopped
collards, and gently heat.
Garnish with croutons.*

Juice Snacks for Any Time of Day

Gingerberry Pops

1 quart blueberries
1-inch slice ginger root
1 medium bunch green
    grapes
3-oz. paper cups
Wooden popsicle sticks

*Push blueberries and ginger
through hopper with grapes.
Pour juice into cups, add
sticks, and freeze.*

Very Berry Freeze

1 large bunch green grapes 1 large bunch red grapes 1 quart blueberries or blackberries	*Juice green grapes. Pour juice into ice cube tray and freeze. Push red grapes and berries through hopper, and pour juice into tall glass. Add frozen grape cubes and garnish with small cluster of grapes.*

Fruit Tea

1 orange, peeled (leave white pithy part) 1 red apple, seeded 1 lime wedge 1 quart water	*Juice fruit. Place juice in saucepan, add water, and gently heat.*

High-Calcium Drink

3 kale leaves Small handful parsley 4–5 carrots, greens removed	*Bunch up kale and parsley, and push through hopper with carrots.*

Ginger Fizz

¼-inch slice ginger root 1 apple, seeded Sparkling water	*Push ginger through hopper with apple. Pour juice into ice-filled glass. Fill glass to top with sparkling water.*

Lemon Spritzer

1 small lemon Sparkling water	*Push lemon through hopper. Pour juice into ice-filled glass. Fill glass to top with sparkling water.*

SUGGESTED MENU FOR BREAKING THE JUICE FAST

DAY ONE

Breakfast

Juice: _____
Fruit or vegetable salad with
  lemon juice dressing
Herbal tea

Mid-Morning Snack

Juice: _____

Lunch

Juice: _____
Harvest Soup
Vegetable salad with lemon
  juice dressing

Mid-Afternoon Snack

Juice: _____
  or herbal tea

Dinner

Juice: _____
Vegetable soup or steamed
  vegetables
Vegetable salad

Bedtime Snack

Juice: _____
  or herbal tea

DAY TWO

Breakfast

Juice: _____
Same as above

Mid-Morning Snack

Juice: _____

Lunch

Juice: _____
Vegetable salad
Brown rice
Vegetable soup

Mid-Afternoon Snack

Juice: _____
  or herbal tea

Dinner

Juice: _____
Vegetable salad with lemon
  juice and olive oil dressing
Baked potato
Baked or broiled fish

Bedtime Snack

Juice: _____
  or herbal tea

THE SENECA INDIAN CLEANSING DIET

This diet is believed to have a different cleansing effect during each of the four days. The first day, the colon is cleansed. The second day, toxins are released along with excess salts and calcium deposits. The third day, the digestive tract is supplied with mineral-rich fiber. And finally, on the fourth day, the blood, lymphatic system, and other organs are nourished with minerals.

SENECA INDIAN CLEANSING DIET GUIDELINES

☐ **Day One: Eat only fruits and their juices.** You may choose from apples, pears, berries, melons, peaches, and cherries.

☐ **Day Two: Drink all the herbal teas you want.** You may choose from raspberry, chamomile, peppermint, and many other varieties.

☐ **Day Three: Eat all the vegetables you desire.** They can be raw, steamed, or cooked in soups.

☐ **Day Four: Make a large soup pot of vegetable broth.** Simmer cauliflower, cabbage, parsley, green pepper, onion, garlic, or any other vegetables. Season with sea salt and vegetable broth cubes. Drink only the broth all day.

THE SEVEN–DAY LIVER-CLEANSING DIET

For this diet, follow the Basic Diet (see page 285), adding the following foods to your daily diet plan.

SEVEN-DAY LIVER-CLEANSING DIET GUIDELINES

□ **Eat this Carrot Salad every day.** Take one cup of very finely shredded carrots or carrot pulp. The carrots should be shredded to a mushy consistency with a food processor or fine grater, or you can use the carrot pulp left over from making carrot juice. If the pulp seems too dry, moisten it with a little carrot juice. Combine 1 tablespoon of olive oil with 1 tablespoon of fresh lemon juice. (You may add more lemon or olive oil, but not less.) Pour over the carrot pulp or grated carrots as a dressing and mix well. If you like, add pineapple or raisins to taste. Eat this salad every day for seven days. If you miss a day, you must begin all over again. This salad is very helpful in cleansing the liver.

□ **Eat one to two cups of Vegetable Broth each day.**

2–3 cups chopped green beans
2–3 cups chopped zucchini
2–3 stalks celery, chopped
1 Tbsp. unsalted butter
1–3 Tbsp. chopped parsley
Season with ginger, cayenne, herbs, garlic, or vegetable broth as desired.

Steam green beans, zucchini, and celery in water until soft, but still green. Put the vegetables in a blender and purée until smooth. The broth should be fairly thick. Add butter and chopped parsley. Season to taste.

□ **Drink two glasses of Green Drink each day.** Make one cup of green juice from any green vegetables. Suggested vegetables include beet tops, spinach, parsley, zucchini, kale, cucumbers, green leafy lettuce, dandelion leaves, collard greens, and wheatgrass. Add to your green drink mixture an equal part of a mild-tasting juice like carrot, apple, tomato, or pineapple. (We don't recommend drinking green juices straight because they are too strong and can be irritating to the throat.) This drink has been used traditionally as an aid for digestion. It is high in chlorophyll, which is said to help detoxify the body and cleanse the blood.

☐ **Drink three ounces of beet juice each day.** If you have more than three ounces per day when you begin the cleansing program, you may cleanse your body a little faster than you want. After the first couple of days, you can increase the amount of beet juice one ounce at a time.

☐ **Take the herb milk thistle each day.** Milk thistle contains some of the most potent liver-cleansing and protecting substances known. The active nutrient in milk thistle, silymarin, enhances liver function and inhibits factors that cause hepatic damage. Silymarin prevents free radical damage through its antioxidant properties. A traditional remedy recommends one tablet with each meal for seven days.

☐ **Avoid all alcohol.**

☐ **Avoid all junk foods and sweets.**

THE SIX-WEEK CLEANSING DIET

This diet is designed to detoxify the body slowly over time. It can be used in conjunction with a one- to five-day juice fast. The goal is to avoid all animal products during this period, as well as refined and processed foods. The following guidelines should be followed closely for maximum benefit. Please note that you may wish to eat more on this temporary cleansing diet because it is low in calories.

SUGGESTED MENU

Breakfast

Juice: _____
Fresh fruit
Cereal with soymilk or juice
Whole wheat or whole rye toast
Herbal tea

Mid-Morning Snack

Juice: _____
  or fresh fruit

Lunch

Salad
Soup
Baked potato
Steamed vegetables
Herbal tea

Mid-Afternoon Snack

Vegetable Juice: _____
Vegetable sticks

Dinner

Vegetarian bean bake
Salad
Soup
Brown rice or millet
Cooked vegetables
Fruit for dessert
Herbal teas

Evening Snack

Juice: _____
Herbal tea

SIX-WEEK CLEANSING DIET GUIDELINES

☐ Beverages

Recommended Foods: Herbal teas such as mint, licorice root, dandelion, nettles, red clover, raspberry, and chamomile. Coffee substitutes such as Pero or Cafix are also permissible.

Foods to Avoid: Alcohol, cocoa, coffee, decaffeinated coffee, milk, and soft drinks.

☐ Bread and Grains

Recommended Foods: Whole wheat, rye, buckwheat, millet, bran, corn, 7-grain, soy, and brown rice. Purchase only whole grains that are preservative free.

Foods to Avoid: White rice, white bread, and blends that contain some white flour. Be aware that white flour is often referred to as wheat flour. If whole grains are used, the label will read "whole wheat flour."

☐ Cereals

Recommended Foods: Oatmeal, brown and wild rice, millet, buckwheat, groats, barley, cornmeal, cracked wheat, and 7-grain.

Foods to Avoid: Cereals that are puffed, flaked, or similarly processed. Also avoid white rice.

☐ Dairy Products

Foods to Avoid: All dairy products. You can substitute soy, almond, or sesame milk for cow's milk. You can substitute soy cheese for cheese made from animal milk.

☐ Eggs

Foods to Avoid: Eggs and all foods that contain eggs.

☐ Fat

Recommended Foods: Cold-pressed or expeller-pressed oils such as olive, safflower, sunflower, sesame, walnut, corn, or soy.

Foods to Avoid: Butter, shortening, margarine, and saturated oils such as coconut and cottonseed. Avoid rancid oils. Make sure all oils are refrigerated after opening.

☐ Meats, Poultry, and Fish

Foods to Avoid: All meats, poultry, and fish.

☐ Legumes

Recommended Foods: Beans, lentils, and split peas.

☐ Vegetables

Recommended Foods: All vegetables, raw, freshly steamed, or cooked in soups. Produce should be organically grown whenever possible. Peel or wash thoroughly all sprayed vegetables. Potatoes should be baked or steamed in their jackets and seasoned with an herbal seasoning or salad dressing. Eat plenty of salads.

Foods to Avoid: Sprayed, canned, frozen, and sulfite-treated vegetables.

☐ Fruit

Recommended Foods: Fresh fruits, organically grown whenever possible. Peel or wash thoroughly all sprayed fruit. Use citrus fruit sparingly. Choose only unsulfured dried fruit.

Foods to Avoid: Sprayed, canned, frozen, and sulfur-dried fruits.

☐ Juices

Recommended Foods: Only freshly made juices. Beet and cabbage are especially cleansing. Drink 4–6 glasses of fresh juice every day. Drink more vegetable juice than fruit juice.

Foods to Avoid: All canned, bottled, and frozen juices.

☐ Nuts

Recommended Foods: Fresh raw nuts. Walnuts, almonds, and pecans are best. Raw nut butters (except peanut butter) are good choices on toast, crackers, and bread.

Foods to Avoid: Peanuts and peanut butter, cashews, Brazil nuts, and pine nuts, as well as roasted and salted nuts of all kinds.

☐ Seeds

Recommended Foods: Raw sunflower, chia, sesame, and pumpkin seeds.

Foods to Avoid: Roasted and salted seeds.

☐ Sprouts

Recommended Foods: All sprouts, such as alfalfa, mung, lentil, radish, and wheatgrass. Add them to salads, sandwiches, and juice drinks.

☐ Desserts

Recommended Foods: Only fresh fruit, stewed fruit, or natural fruit gelatin made with agar. Sweeten only with honey, pure maple syrup, fruit juice concentrate, or brown rice syrup.

Foods to Avoid: Canned or frozen fruit, commercial gelatin desserts, pastries, cakes, pies, cookies, ice cream, custard, candy, and so forth.

Weight-Loss Diets

THE QUICK WEIGHT-LOSS DIET

This weight-loss diet is designed for people who have a moderate amount of weight to lose—approximately five to thirty pounds. It is not intended for the person who is extremely overweight unless supervision is provided by a health professional.

The concept is simple. Drink juice throughout the day and eat a sensible meal with your family in the evening. Or have your meal at noon and your juice for dinner! Many people report that they just aren't hungry on this diet because the juices are so filling and satisfying. Cherie's husband lost eighteen pounds on this diet and has successfully kept the weight off. He stated that he didn't feel hungry the entire time, and that he had more energy than usual.

People often say that they look five to ten years younger on this diet as well. This is not surprising, since these juices are packed with anti-aging nutrients such as vitamin C and beta-carotene. This is the type of diet that sends thousands of people to famous health spas around the world for the weight loss and the "face lift," as well.

If you wish to lose only a moderate amount of weight, you should be able to safely on this diet until you have reached your goal. But, if you experience any symptoms that concern you, discontinue the diet and seek professional medical help. Also, if you have special health challenges, always seek medical advice before starting a weight-loss diet.

SUGGESTED MENU

The following menu includes several recipe names to give you some idea of how to get started. For these juice drink recipes and many more, see "Recipes for Juice Fast" on page 303.

Breakfast

Energy Shake or Pink Morning Tonic

Mid-Morning Snack

Ginger Hopper or Waldorf Salad

Lunch

Potassium Broth or Garden Salad Special

Mid-Afternoon Snack

Cherie's Cleansing Cocktail or Zippy Spring Tonic

Happy Hour Cocktail

Berry Cantaloupe Shake or Waldorf Salad

Dinner

Salad
Oil and vinegar dressing
Steamed vegetables
Brown rice
Broiled or baked fish
Fruit dessert
Herbal tea

Bedtime Snack

Evening Regulator (see page 103), Waldorf Salad, or chamomile tea

THE LONG-TERM WEIGHT-LOSS DIET

This is not a diet but rather a way of eating. If you have over thirty pounds to loose, read the OVERWEIGHT/OBESITY section in Part Two. It is very important that you start slowly. Permanent weight loss involves many changes in your lifestyle, and a change in eating habits is just one of them. Follow the Basic Diet (see page 285), at first eating as much as you desire from the allowed foods. Together with your exercise program, this will result in a slow, steady weight loss. Don't bother to get on a scale during this breaking-in period; just let your body and mind adjust. When you feel ready, start to cut back on portion size. For three days, measure everything you eat or drink to determine exactly how much you are consuming. This may be a surprise. Overestimating portion size is a common problem that you can learn to overcome. Write down how you are feeling when you eat. Many people discover that they eat more when they are under emotional or psychological stress. To learn more about weight loss, read one of the books in the "Overweight/Obesity" section of the reference list (see page 341).

SUGGESTED MENU

Breakfast

Juice: _____
Whole grain waffle
Nonfat yogurt
Green tea
Apple

Mid-Morning Snack

1 apple

Lunch

Juice: _____
Vegetable soup
Garden salad with 1 Tbsp.
  low-fat dressing
Whole grain roll

Dinner

Juice: _____
Baked skinless chicken
Brown rice
Yellow vegetable
Green vegetable

Evening Snack

3 cups air-popped popcorn

Suggested Reading List

Balch, James F; Balch, Phyllis A. *Prescription for Nutritional Healing.* Avery Publishing Group, Inc., Garden City Park, New York, 1990.

Carper, Jean. *The Food Pharmacy.* Bantam Books, New York, 1988.

Chaitow, Leon. *Candida Albicans.* Thorsons Publishing, Inc., Rochester, Vermont, 1987.

Chelf, Vicki Rae. *Cooking With the Right Side of the Brain.* Avery Publishing Group, Inc., Garden City Park, New York, 1991.

Colbin, Annemarie. *Food and Healing.* Ballantine Books, New York, 1986.

Connor, Sonja L.; Connor, William E. *The New American Diet.* Fireside, New York, 1986.

Crook, William G. *Tracking Down the Hidden Food Allergy.* Professional Books, Jackson, Tennessee, 1980.

Crook, William G. *The Yeast Connection,* Second Edition. Professional Books, Jackson, Tennessee, 1984.

Fink, John M. *Third Opinion.* Avery Publishing Group, Inc., Garden City Park, New York, 1988.

Forbes, Alec. *The Famous Bristol Detox Diet.*, Keats Publishing, Inc., New Canaan, Connecticut, 1984.

Gerson, Max. *A Cancer Therapy.* Gerson Institute, Bonita, California, 1958.

Goldbeck, Nikki; Goldbeck, David. *American Wholefood Cuisine.* New American Library, New York, 1983.

Goldbeck, Nikki; Goldbeck, David. *The Goldbeck's Guide to Good Food.* New American Library, New York, 1987.

Howell, Edward. *Enzyme Nutrition.* Avery Publishing Group, Inc., Garden City Park, New York, 1985.

Hunt, Douglas. *No More Cravings.* Warner Books, New York, 1987.

Jensen, Bernard. *Foods That Heal.* Avery Publishing Group, Inc., Garden City Park, New York, 1988.

Jensen, Bernard. *Tissue Cleansing Through Bowel Management.* Bernard Jensen, Escondido, California, 1981.

Kenton, Leslie; Kenton, Sussanah. *Raw Energy.* Century Publishing, London, 1984.

Kushi, Michio. *The Cancer Prevention Diet.* St. Martin's Press, New York, 1983.

Kushi, Michio. *The Macrobiotic Approach to Cancer,* Second Edition. Avery Publishing Group, Inc., Garden City Park, New York, 1991.

Lieberman, Shari; Bruning, Nancy. *The Real Vitamin and Mineral Book.* Avery Publishing Group, Inc., Garden City Park, New York, 1990.

Mabey, Richard. *The New Age Herbalist.* Collier Books, New York, 1988.

Murray, Michael; Pizzorno, Joseph. *Encyclopedia of Natural Medicine.* Prima Publishing, Rocklin, California, 1990.

Pelletier, Kenneth R. *Mind as Healer, Mind as Slayer.* Dell Publishing, New York, 1977.

Schwartz, Bob. *Diets Don't Work.* Breakthrough Publishing, Houston, 1982.

Smith, Nathan J.; Worthington-Roberts, Bonnie. *Food for Sport.* Bull Publishing Company, Palo Alto, California, 1989.

Stoff, Jesse A.; Pellegrino, Charles R. *Chronic Fatigue Syndrome.* Macmillan Publishing Co., New York, 1988.

Walker, Norman. *Colon Health: The Key to a Vibrant Life.* Walker Press, Prescott, Arizona, 1979.

Weinberger, Stanley. *Healing Within.* Colon Health Center, Larkspur, California, 1988.

Wigmore, Ann. *Hippocrates Live Food Program.* Hippocrates Press, Boston, 1984.

Wigmore, Ann. *The Wheatgrass Book.* Avery Publishing Group, Inc., Garden City Park, New York, 1985.

Yntema, Sharon. *Vegetarian Baby.* McBooks Press, Ithaca, NY, 1980.

References

PART ONE

Kenton, L; Kenton, S. *Raw Energy.* London: Century Publishing, 1984.

Kozora, E.J. *Nutritional Guidelines.* Seattle: American Holistic Medical Association, 1987.

Walker, N.W. *Fresh Vegetable and Fruit Juices.* Prescott, AZ: Norwalk Press, 1970.

PART TWO

Acne

Allen, B.R. Essential fatty acids of the n-6 series in acne and psoriasis; in Harrobin, D.F., Ed.: *Omega-6 Essential Fatty Acids Pathophysiology and Roles in Clinical Medicine.* New York: Alan R. Liss, 1990.

Arbesman, H. Letter to the Editor. *N. Engl. J. Med.* 322(8):558, February 1990.

Ayres, S.; Mihan, R. Acne vulgaris: therapy directed at pathophysiological defects. *Cutis.* 28:2–4, 1981.

Callaghan, T.J. The effect of folic acid on seborrheic dermatitis. *Cutis.* 3:583–588, 1967.

Horrobin, D.F. Essential fatty acids in clinical dermatology. *J. Am. Acad. Derm.* 20:1045–1053, 1989.

Kader, M.M.; Hafiez A.A.; et al. Glucose tolerance in blood and skin of patients with acne vulgaris. *Indian J. Derm.* 22(4):139–149, 1977.

Kaufman, W.F. The diet and acne. *Arch. Derm.* 119:276, 1983.

Kinsella, J.E. Dietary polyunsaturated fatty acids affect inflammatory, immune functions. *The Nutrition Report* 8(10):73–80, October 1990.

Kligman, A.M.; Mills, O.H.; et al. Oral Vitamin A in acne vulgaris. *Int. J. Derm.* 20:278–285, 1981.

McCarty, M. High-chromium yeast for acne? *Med. Hypoth.* 14:307–310, 1984.

Michaelsson, G.; Edquvist, L.E. Erythrocyte glutathione peroxidase activity in acne vulgaris and the effect of selenium and vitamin E treatment. *Acta. Derm. Venereol.* (Stockh.) 64:9–14, 1984.

Michaelsson, G.; Juhlin, L.; et al. Effects of oral zinc and vitamin A in acne. *Arch. Derm.* 113:31–36, 1977.

Pohit, J.; Saha, K.C.; et al. Zinc status of acne vulgaris patients. *J. Applied Nutr.* 37(1):18–25, 1985.

Robberts, C. Letter to the Editor. *N. Engl. J. Med.* 322(8):558, February, 1990.

Rosenberg, E.W. Acne diet reconsidered. *Arch. Derm.* 117:193–195, 1981.

Snider, B.L.; Dieteman, D.F. Pyridoxine therapy for premenstrual acne flare. *Arch. Derm.* 110:130–131, 1974.

Age Spots

Balch, J.; Balch, P. *Prescription for Nutritional Healing.* Garden City Park, NY: Avery Publishing Group, Inc., 1990.

Clark, L. *Secrets of Health and Beauty.* New York: Pyramid Books, 1970.

Aging

Cutler, R.G. Antioxidants and aging. *Am. J. Clin. Nutr.* 53:373S–379S, 1991.

Cutler, R.G. Peroxide-producing potential of tissues: inverse correlation with longevity of mammalian species. *Prox. Natil. Acad. Sci.* 81:7627–7631, 1984.

Hayflick, L. The cell biology of human aging. *N. Engl. J. Med.* 295:302–308, 1976.

Jones, E., et al. Quercetin, flavonoids and the life-span of mice. *Exp. Gerontology* 17(3):213–217, 1982.

Kenton, L.; Kenton, S. *Raw Energy.* London: Century Publishing, 1984.

Kuhnau, J. The flavonoids: a class of semi-essential food components: their role in human nutrition. *Wld. Rev. Nutr. Diet.* 24:117–191, 1976.

Murray, M.; Pizzorno, J. *Encyclopedia of Natural Medicine.* Rocklin, CA: Prima Publishing, 1990.

Schneider, E.L., et al. Life extension. *N. Engl. J. Med.* 312:159–168, 1985.

Allergies

Amella, M., et al. Inhibition of mast cell histamine release by flavonoids and bioflavonoids. *Planta Medica* 51:16–20, 1985.

Clemetson, C.A. Histamine and ascorbic acid in human blood. *J. Nutr.* 110(4):662–668, 1980.

Folkers, K., et al. Biochemical evidence for a deficiency of vitamin B_6 in subjects reacting to monosodium-L-glutamate by the Chinese restaurant syndrome. *Biochem. Biophys. Res. Commun.* 100L972–977, 1980.

Kamimura, M. Anti-inflammatory activity of vitamin E. *J. Vitaminol.* 18(4):204–209, 1972.

Kuvaeva, L., et al. The microecology of the gastrointestinal tract and the immunological status under food allergy. *Nahrung* 28(6–7):689–693, 1984.

Papaioannou, R., et al. Sulfite sensitivity—unrecognized threat: is molybdenum the cause? *J. Orthomol. Psychiat.* 105–110, 1984.

Pastorello, E., et al. Evaluation of allergic etiology in perennial rhinitis. *Ann. Allergy* 55:854–856, 1984.

Simon, S.W. Vitamin B_{12} therapy in allergy and chronic dermatoses. *J. Allergy* 2:183–185, 1951.

Alzheimer's Disease

Abalan, F., et al. B_{12} deficiency in presenile dementia. *Biol. Psychiatry* 20:1247–1251, 1985.

Balch, J.; Balch, P. *Prescription for Nutritional Healing.* Garden City Park, NY: Avery Publishing Group, Inc., 1990.

Burnet, F.M. A possible role of zinc in the pathology of dementia. *Lancet* i:186–188, 1981.

Candy, J.M., et al. Aluminosilicates and senile plaque formation in Alzheimer's disease. *Lancet* i:354–357, 1986.

Murray, M.; Pizzorno, J. *Encyclopedia of Natural Medicine.* Rocklin, CA: Prima Publishing, 1990.

Nordstrom, J.W. Trace mineral nutrition in the elderly. *Am. J. Clin. Nutr.* 36:788–795, 1982.

Anemia

Borch-Johnsen, B.; Meltzer H.; et al. Bioavailability of daily low dose iron supplements in menstruating women with low iron stores. *Eur. J. Clin.* 44:29–34, 1990.

Krause, M.V.; Mahan, L.K. *Food, Nutrition and Diet Therapy.* Philadelphia: W.B. Saunders, 1984.

Murray, M.; Pizzorno, J. *Encyclopedia of Natural Medicine.* Rocklin, CA: Prima Publishing, 1990.

Arthritis / Osteoarthritis

Bland, J.W., et al. Osteoarthritis: A review of the cell biology involved and evidence of reversibility. Management rationally related to known genesis and pathophysiology. *Seminars in Arthritis & Rhem.* 14(2):106–133, 1984.

Di Padova, C. S-adenosylmethionine in the treatment of osteoarthritis. Review of clinical studies. *Am. J. Med.* 83(5A):60–65, 1987.

Huskisson, E.C., et al. Orgotein in osteoarthritis of the knee joint. *Eur.*

J. Rheumatol. Inflammation 4:212, 1981.

Kaufman, W. The use of vitamin therapy to reverse certain concomitants of aging. *J. Am. Geriatr. Soc.* 3:927, 1955.

Kuhanu, J. The flavonoids. A class of semi-essential food components: their role in human nutrition. *World Review Nutrition and Dietetics.* 24:117–191, 1976.

Machtey, I., et al. Tocopherol in osteoarthritis: a controlled pilot study. *J. Am. Geriatr. Soc.*, 1978.

Nelson, M.N., et al. *Proc. Soc. Exp. Biol.* 73:31, 1950.

Palmblad, J., et al. Antirheumatic effects of fasting. *Rheumatic Dis. Clinic of N. Am.: Nutr. & Rheumatic Dis.* 17(2):351–361, May 1991.

Arthritis / Rheumatoid Arthritis

Barton-Wright, E.C., et al. The pantothenic acid metabolism of rheumatoid arthritis. *Lancet* 2:862–863, 1963.

Chayen, J., et al. The effect of experimentally induced redox changes on human rheumatoid and non-rheumatoid synovial tissue in vitro. *Beitr. Path. Bd.* 149:127, 1973.

Cohen, A., et al. Bromelains therapy in rheumatoid arthritis. *Pennsyl. Med. J.* 67:27–30, June 1964.

Goebel, K.M., et al. Intrasynovial orgotein therapy in rheumatoid arthritis. *Lancet* 1:1015–1017, 1981.

Hartung, E.F., et al. Gastric acidity in chronic arthritis. *Ann. Int. Med.* 9:252–257, 1935.

Kremer, J.M., et al. Effect of manipulation of dietary fatty acids on clinical manifestations of rheumatoid arthritis. *Lancet* 1:184–187, 1985.

Lucas, C., et al. Dietary fats aggravate rheumatoid arthritis. *Clin. Res.* 29(4):754A, 1981.

Mullen, A., et al. The metabolism of ascorbic acid in rheumatoid arthritis. *Proc. Nutr. Sci.* 35:8A–9A, 1976.

Niedermeier, W. Concentration and chemical state of copper in synovial fluid and blood serum of patients with rheumatoid arthritis. *Ann. Rheum. Dis.* 24:544, 1965.

Neidermeier, W., et al. Trace metal composition of synovial fluid and blood serum of patients with rheumatoid arthritis. *J. Chron. Dis.* 23–527–36, 1971.

Palmblad, J., et al. Antirheumatic effects on fasting. *Rheumatic Dis. Clinic of N. Am.: Nutr. & Rheumatic Dis.* 17(2):351–361, 1991.

Pandey, S.P., et al. Zinc in rheumatoid arthritis. *Indian Med. Res.* 81:618–620, 1985.

Panush, R.S., et al. Food-induced (allergic) arthritis. *Arthritis Rheum.* 29(2):220–226, 1986.

Skoldstam, L. Fasting and vegan diet in rheumatoid arthritis. *Scand. J. Rheumatol.* 15(2):219–221, 1987.

Tarp, U., et al. Low selenium level in severe rheumatoid arthritis. *Scand. J. Rheumatol.* 14:97, 1985.

Woldenberg, S.C. The treatment of arthritis with colloidal sulphur. *J. Southern Med. Assoc.* 28:875–881, 1935.

Asthma

Anderson, R., et al. Ascorbic acid in bronchial asthma. *S. A. Med. J.* 63:649–652, 1983.

Bray, G.W. The hypochlorhydria of asthma in childhood. *Quart. J. Med.* 24:181–197, 1931.

Freedman, B.J. A diet free from additives in the management of allergic disease. *Clin. Allergy* 7:417–421, 1977.

Grosch, W., et al. Co-oxidation of carotenes requires one soybean lipoxygenase. *Biochem. Biophys. Acta* 575:439–445, 1979.

Lindahl, O., et al. Vegan regimen with reduced medication in the treatment of bronchial asthma. *J. Asthma* 22(1):45–55, 1985.

Lundberg, J.M., et al. Capsicum-induced desensitization of airway mucosa to cigarette smoke, mechanical and chemical irritants. *Nature* 302:251–253, 1983.

McCarty, M. Can dietary selenium reduce leukotriene production? *Med. Hypoth.* 13:45–50, 1984.

Murray, M.; Pizzorno, J. *Encyclopedia of Natural Medicine.* Rocklin, CA: Prima Publishing, 1990.

Ogle, K.A., et al. Children with allergic rhinitis and/or bronchial asthma treated with elimination diet: a five-year follow-up. *Am. Allergy* 44:273–278, 1980.

Panganamala, R.V., et al. The effects of vitamin E on arachidonic acid metabolism. *Ann. N.Y. Acad. Sci.* 393–376–91, 1982.

Reynolds, R.D., et al. Depressed plasma pyridoxal phosphate concentrates in adult asthmatics. *Am. J. Clin. Nutr.* 41:684–688, 1985.

Stevenson, D.D., et al. Sensitivity to ingested metabisulfites in asthmatic subjects. *J. Allergy Clin. Immunol.* 68:26–32, 1981.

Tan, Y., et al. Aspirin-induced asthma in children. *Ann. Allery* 48:1–5, 1982.

Vanderhoek, J., et al. Inhibition of fatty acid lipoxygenases by onion and garlic oils. Evidence of mechanism by which these oils inhibit platelet aggregation. *Bioch. Pharmacol.* 29:3169–3173, 1980.

Atherosclerosis

Brattstrom, L.E., et al. Folic acid responsive postmenopausal homocysteinemia. *Metabolism* 34(11):1073–1077, 1985.

Burch, G.A., et al. The importance of magnesium deficiency in cardiovascular disease. *Am. Heart J.* 94:649–657, 1977.

Eichner, E.R. Alcohol versus exercise for coronary protection. *Am. J. Med.* 79(2):231–240, 1985.

Karl, J., et al. Coffee, tea and plasma cholesterol: the Jerusalem lipid research clinic prevalence study. *Brit. Med. J.* 291(6497):699–704, 1985.

Klevay, L.M. Dietary copper: a powerful determinant of cholesterolemia. *Med. Hypoth.* 24:111–119, 1987.

Nordrehaug, J., et al. Serum potassium concentration as a risk factor of ventricular arrhythmias early in acute mycardial infarction. *Circulation* 71(4):645–691, 1985.

Reiser, S. Effect of dietary sugars on metabolic risk factors associated with heart disease. *Nutr. & Health,* 1985.

Reynaud, S., et al. Protective effects of dietary calcium and magnesium on platelet function and atherosclerosis in rabbits fed saturated fat. *Atherosclerosis* 47:187–198, 1983.

Rosenthal, M.B., et al. Effects of a high-complex-carbohydrate, low fat, low cholesterol diet on serum lipids and estradiol. *Am. J. Med.* 78:23–27, 1985.

Serfontein, W.J., et al. Plasma pyridoxal-5-phosphate level as risk index for coronary artery disease. *Atherosclerosis* 55:357–361, 1985.

Simonoff, M., et al. Low plasma chromium in patients with coronary artery and heart diseases. *Biological Trace Element Res.* 6:431, 1984.

Steiner, M. Effect of alpha-tocopherol administration on platelet function in man. *Thromb. Haemost.* 49(2):73–77, 1983.

Turley, S., et al. Role of ascorbic acid in the regulation of cholesterol metabolism and the pathogenesis of atherosclerosis. *Atherosclerosis* 24:1–18, 1976.

Virtamo, J., et al. Serum selenium and the risk of coronary heart disease and stroke. *Am. J. Epidemiology* 122:276–282, 1985.

Backache

Bhathena, S., et al. Decreased plasma enkephalins in copper deficiency in man. *Am. J. Clin. Nutr.* 43:42–46, 1986.

Boublik, J.H., et al. Coffee contains potent opiate receptor binding activity. *Nature* 301:246–248, 1983.

Murray, M.; Pizzorno, J. *Encyclopedia of Natural Medicine.* Rocklin, CA: Prima Publishing, 1990.

Walsh, N.E., et al. Analgesic effectiveness of D-phenylalanine in chronic pain patients. *Arch. Phys. Med. Rehabil.* 67(7):436–439, 1986.

Bladder Infection

Elnima, E.I., et al. The antimicrobial activity of garlic and onion extracts. *Pharmazie* 38:747–748, 1983.

Murray, M.; Pizzorno, J. *Encyclopedia of Natural Medicine.*

Rocklin, CA: Prima Publishing, 1990.

Sobota, A.E. Inhibition of bacterial adherence by cranberry juice: potential use for the treatment of urinary tract infections. *J. Urology* 131:1013–1016, 1984.

Bronchitis

Balch, J.; Balch, P. *Prescription for Nutritional Healing.* Garden City Park, NY: Avery Publishing Group, Inc., 1990.

Escott-Stump, S. *Nutrition and Diagnosis-Related Care*, Second Edition. Philadelphia: Lea & Febiger, 1988.

Murray, M.; Pizzorno, J. *Encyclopedia of Natural Medicine.* Rocklin, CA: Prima Publishing, 1990.

Bruising

Cragin, R.B. The use of bioflavonoids in the prevention and treatment of athletic injuries. *Med. Times* 90:529–530, 1962.

Garbor, M. Pharmacologic effect of flavonoids on blood vessels. *Angiologica*, 1972.

Bursitis

Biskind, M.S., et al. The use of citrus flavonoids in infection II. *Am. J. Digest Dis.* 24:41–45, 1955.

Kim, J., et al. The effect of vitamin E on the healing of gingival wounds in rats. *J. Periodontal.* 54:305–308, 1983.

Klemes, I.S. Vitamin B_{12} in acute subdeltoid bursitis. *Indust. Med. & Surg.*, 1957.

Krause, M.; Mahan, L. *Food, Nutrition and Diet Therapy.* Philadelphia: W.B. Saunders, 1984.

Murray, M.; Pizzorno, J. *Encyclopedia of Natural Medicine.*

Rocklin, CA: Prima Publishing, 1990.

Cancer

Belman, S. Onion and garlic oil inhibit tumor growth. *Carcinogenesis* 4(8):1063–1065, 1983.

Berry, I.R. The anti-cancer vitamin beta-carotene. *Total Health* 12(3):55(1), June 1990.

Block, G. Vitamin C and cancer prevention: the epidemiologic evidence. *Am. J. Clin. Nutr.* 53:270S–282S, 1991.

Borgeson, C.E., et al. Effects of dietary fish oils on human mammary carcinoma and on lipid metabolizing enzymes. *Lipids* 24:290–295, 1989.

Diplock, A. Antioxidant nutrients and disease prevention: an overview. *Am. J. Clin. Nutr.* 53:189S–193S, 1991.

DiSogra, C.; Groll, L. *Nutrition and Cancer Prevention.* Department of Social and Health Services, 1981.

Draper, H.H., et al. Micronutrients and cancer prevention: are the RDA's adequate? *Free Radical Biology and Medicine* 3:203–207, 1987.

Garland, C., et al. Dietary vitamin D and calcium and risk of colorectal cancer. A 19-year prospective study for men. *Lancet* 1:3–7–9, 1985.

Garwell, H.S. Potential role of B-carotene in prevention of oral cancer. *Am. J. Clinc. Nutr.* 53:294S–297S, 1991.

Lippman, S.M., et al. Vitamin A derivatives in the prevention and treatment of cancer. *J. Am. Coll. Nutr.* 7(4):269–284, 1988.

Prasod, K.N., et al. Vitamin E increases the growth inhibitory and differentiating effects of tumor therapeutic agents on neuroblastoma and glioma cell in culture. *Proc. Soc. Exp. Biol. Med.* 164(2): 158–163, 1980.

Pryor, W.A. The antioxidant nutrients and disease prevention—what do we know and what do we need to find out? *Am. J. Clin. Nutr.* 53:391S–393S, 1991.

Watson, R.R., et al. Selenium and vitamins A, E and C: nutrients with cancer prevention properties. *J. Am. Diet. Assoc.* 86(4):505–510, 1986.

Candidiasis

Abe, F., et al. Experimental candidiasis in liver injury. *Mycopathologia* 100:37–42, 1987.

Amer, M., et al. The effect of aqueous garlic extract on the growth of dermatophytes. *Int. J. Dermatol.*, 1980.

Collins, E.B., et al. Inhibition of Candida albicans by Lactobacillus acidophilus. *J. Dairy Sci.* 63:830–832, 1980.

Crook, W.G. *The Yeast Connection*, Second Edition. Jackson, TN: Professional Books, 1984.

Galland, L. Nutrition and candidiasis. *J. Orthomol. Psychiatry* 15:50–60, 1985.

Lorenzani, S. *Candida: A Twentieth Century Disease.* New Canaan, CT: Keats Publishing, 1986.

Murray, M.; Pizzorno, J. *Encyclopedia of Natural Medicine.* Rocklin, CA: Prima Publishing, 1990.

Ransberger, K. Enzyme treatment of immune complex diseases. *Arthritis Rheuma.* 8:16–19m, 1986.

Canker Sores

Balch, J.; Balch, P. *Prescription for Nutritional Healing.* Garden City Park, NY: Avery Publishing Group, Inc., 1990.

Hay, K.D., et al. The use of an elimination diet in the treatment of recurrent aphthous ulceration of the oral cavity. *Oral Surg.* 57:504–507, 1984.

Little, J.W. Food allergens and basophil histamine release in recurrent aphthous stomatitis. *Oral Surg.* 54:388–395, 1982.

Ship, I.I., et al. Recurrent aphthous ulcers. *Am. J. Med.* 32:32–43, 1962.

Wray, D. Gluten-sensitive recurrent aphthous stomatitis. *Dig. Dis. Sci.* 26–737–40, 1981.

Wray, D., et al. Recurrent aphthae: treatment with vitamin B_{12}, folic acid, and iron. *Brit. Med. J.* 2:490–493, 1975.

Cataracts

Atkinson, D. Malnutrition as an etiological factor in senile cataract. *Eye, Ear, Nose and Throat Monthly* 31:79–83, 1952.

Balch, J.; Balch, P. *Prescription for Nutritional Healing.* Garden City Park, NY: Avery Publishing Group, Inc., 1990.

Bhat, K. Plasma calcium and trace metals in human subjects with mature cataract. *Nutr. Rep. Int.* 37:157–163, 1988.

Bouton, S. Vitamin C and the aging eye. *Arch. Int. Med.* 63:930–945, 1939.

Burton, G., et al. Beta-carotene: an unusual type of lipid antioxidant. *Science* 224:569–573, 1984.

Haranaka, R., et al. Pharmacological action of Hachimijiogan (Baweiwan) on the metabolism of aged subjects. *Am. J. Chinese Med.* 24:59–67, 1986.

Jacques, P.F., et al. Antioxidant status in persons with and without senile cataract. *Arch. Opthal.* 106:337–340, 1988.

Murray, M.; Pizzorno, J. *Encyclopedia of Natural Medicine.* Rocklin, CA: Prima Publishing, 1990.

Rathbun, W., et al. Glutathione metabolic pathway as a scavening system in the lens. *Ophthal. Res.* 11:172–176, 1979.

Shalka, H., et al. Cataracts and riboflavin deficiency. *Am. J. Clin. Nutr.* 34:861–863, 1981.

Swanson, A., et al. Elemental analysis in normal and cataractuous human lens tissue. *Biochem. Biophy. Res. Comm.* 45:1488–1496, 1971.

Taylor, A. Associations between nutrition and cataract. *Nutr.* Reviews 47(8):225–235, 1989.

Varma, S.D. Scientific basis for medical therapy of cataracts by antioxidants. *Am. J. Clin. Nutr.* 53-335S–45S, 1991.

Whanger, P., et al. Effects of selenium, chromium and antioxidants on growth, eye cataracts, plasma cholesterol and blood glucose in selenium deficient, vitamin E supplemented rats. *Nutr. Rep. Int.* 12:345–358, 1975.

Cellulite

Kenton, L.; Kenton, S. *Raw Energy.* London: Century Publishing, 1984.

Murray, M.; Pizzorno, J. *Encyclopedia of Natural Medicine.* Rocklin, CA: Prima Publishing, 1990.

Scherwitz, C., et al. So-called cellulite. *J. Dermatol. Surg. Oncol.* 4:230–234, 1978.

Cholesterolemia

Altschule, M.D. A tale of two lipids. Cholesterol and Eicosapentaneoic acid. *Chest* 89(4):601–602, 1986.

Anderson, J.W., et al. Dietary fiber: hyperlipidemia, hypertension, and coronary heart disease. *Am. J. Gastroenterology* 81(10):907–919, 1986.

Balch, J.; Balch, P. *Prescription for Nutritional Healing.* Garden City Park, NY: Avery Publishing Group, Inc., 1990.

Bordia, A.K., et al. Effect of the essential oils of garlic and onion on alimentary hyperlipidemia. *Atherosclerosis* 21:15–19, 1975.

Carper, J. *The Food Pharmacy.* New York: Bantam Books, 1988.

Connor, S.; Connor, W. *The New American Diet.* New York: Fireside, 1986.

Degroot, A.P., et al. Cholesterol-lowering effect of rolled oats. *Lancet* 2:203–204, 1983.

Giri, J., et al. Effect of ginger on serum cholesterol levels. *Ind. J. Nutr. Diet.* 21:433–436, 1984.

Horrobin, D.F. A new concept of lifestyle-related cardiovascular disease: the importance of interactions between cholesterol, essential fatty acids, prostaglandin E1 and thromboxane A2. *Med. Hypoth.* 6:785–800, 1980.

Lo, G.S., et al. Soy fiber improves lipid and carbohydrate metabolism in primary hyperlipidemic subjects. *Atherosclerosis* 62:239–248, 1986.

Owren, P.A. Coronary thrombosis: its mechanisms and possible prevention by linoleic acid. *Ann. Int. Med.* 63(2):167–184.

Robertson, J., et al. The effect of raw carrot on serum lipids and colon function. *Am. J. Clin. Nutr.* 32(9):1889–1892, 1979.

Sable-Amplis, R., et al. Further studies on the cholesterol-lowering effect of apple in humans:

biochemical mechanisms involved. *Nutr. Res.* 3:325–328, 1983.

Sambaiah, K., et al. Hypocholesterolemic effect of red pepper and capsaicin. *Indian Journal of Experimental Biology*, 1980.

Sincalir, H.M. Deficiency of essential fatty acids and atherosclerosis, etcetera. Letters to the Editor. *Lancet* 381–383, April 7, 1956.

Werbach, M. *Nutritional Influences on Illness*. Tarzana, CA: Third Line Press, Inc., 1987.

Whitney, E.; Cataldo, C.; Rolfes, S. *Understanding Normal and Clinical Nutrition*. New York: West Publishing Co., 1983.

Chronic Fatigue Syndrome

Alexander, M., et al. Oral beta-carotene can increase the number of OKT4+ cells in human blood. *Immunology Letters* 9:221–224, 1985.

Balch, J.; Balch, P. *Prescription for Nutritional Healing*. Garden City Park, NY: Avery Publishing Group, Inc., 1990.

Beisel, W., et al. Single-nutrient effects of immunologic functions. *J.A.M.A.* 245:53–58, 1981.

Murray, M.; Pizzorno, J. *Encyclopedia of Natural Medicine*. Rocklin, CA: Prima Publishing, 1990.

Schwerdt, P., et al. Effect of ascorbic acid on rhinovirus replication in W1-38 cells. *Proc. Soc. Exp. Biol. Med.* 148:1237–1243, 1975.

Straus, S.E., et al. Persisting illness and fatigue in adults with evidence of Epstein-Barr virus infection. *Ann. Int. Med.* 102:7–16, 1985.

Circulation Problems

Balch, J.; Balch, P. *Prescription for Nutritional Healing*. Garden City

Park, NY: Avery Publishing Group, Inc., 1990.

Colitis

Balch, J.; Balch, P. *Prescription for Nutritional Healing*. Garden City Park, NY: Avery Publishing Group, Inc., 1990.

Escott-Stump, S. *Nutrition and Diagnosis-Related Care*. Philadelphia: Lea & Febiger, 1988.

Krause, M.; Mahan, L. *Food, Nutrition and Diet Therapy*. Philadelphia: W.B. Saunders, 1984.

Mabey, R. *The New Age Herbalist*. New York: Collier Books, 1988.

Murray, M.; Pizzorno, J. *Encyclopedia of Natural Medicine*. Rocklin, CA: Prima Publishing, 1990.

Shils, M.; Young, V. *Modern Nutrition in Health and Disease*. Philadelphia: Lea & Febiger, 1988.

Common Cold

Alexander, M., et al. Oral beta-carotene can increase the number of OKT4+ cells in human blood. *Immunology Letters* 9:221–224, 1985.

Anderson, T., et al. Vitamin C and the common cold: a double blind trial. *Can. Med. Assoc. J.* 107:503–508, 1972.

Balch, J.; Balch, P. *Prescription for Nutritional Healing*. Garden City Park, NY: Avery Publishing Group, Inc., 1990.

Eby, G., et al. Reduction in duration of common colds by zinc gluconate lozenges in a double-blind study. *Antimicrob. Agents Chemother.* 25:20–24, 1984.

Mabey, R. *The New Age Herbalist*. New York: Collier Books, 1988.

Murray, M.; Pizzorno, J. *En-cyclopedia of Natural Medicine.* Rocklin, CA: Prima Publishing, 1990.

Sanchez, A., et al. Role of sugars in human neutrophilic phagocytosis. *Am. J. Clin. Nutr.* 26:1180–1184, 1973.

Constipation

Balch, J.; Balch, P. *Prescription for Nutritional Healing.* Garden City Park, NY: Avery Publishing Group, Inc., 1990.

Boetz, M.I., et al. Neurologic disorders responsive to folic acid therapy. *Can. Med. Assoc. J.* 14:217, 1976.

Escott-Stump, S. *Nutrition and Diagnosis-Related Care.* Philadelphia: Lea & Febiger, 1988.

Franklin, J.F. Treatment of chronic constipation. Questions and answers. *J.A.M.A.* 256(6):652, 1986.

Gay, L.P. Gastrointestinal allergy. *J. Missouri Med. Assoc.* 29:7–10, 1932.

Krause, M.; Mahan, L. *Food, Nutrition and Diet Therapy.* Philadelphia: W.B. Saunders, 1984.

Murray, M.; Pizzorno, J. *En-cyclopedia of Natural Medicine.* Rocklin, CA: Prima Publishing, 1990.

Weinberger, S. *Healing Within.* Larkspur, CA: Colon Health Center, 1988.

Cravings

Hunt, D. *No More Cravings.* New York: Warner Books, 1987.

Murray, M.; Pizzorno, J. *En-cyclopedia of Natural Medicine.* Rocklin, CA: Prima Publishing, 1990.

Crohn's Disease

Balch, J.; Balch, P. *Prescription for Nutritional Healing.* Garden City Park, NY: Avery Publishing Group, Inc., 1990.

Escott-Stump, S. *Nutrition and Diagnosis-Related Care.* Philadelphia: Lea & Febiger, 1988.

Heaton, K.W., et al. Treatment of Crohn's disease with an unrefined-carbohydrate, fibre-rich diet. *Brit. Med. J.* 279:764–766, 1979.

Hodges, P., et al. Vitamin and iron intake in patients with Crohn's disease. *J. Am. Diet. Assoc.* 84(1):52–58, 1984.

Murray, M.; Pizzorno, J. *En-cyclopedia of Natural Medicine.* Rocklin, CA: Prima Publishing, 1990.

O'Morain, C., et al. Elemental diet in acute Crohn's disease. *Arch. Dis. Childhood* 53:44, 1983.

Siegel, J. Inflammatory bowel disease: another possible facet of allergic diathesis. *Ann. Allergy* 47:92–94, 1981.

Depression

Balch, J.; Balch P. *Prescription for Nutritional Healing.* Garden City Park, NY: Avery Publishing Group, Inc., 1990.

Carney, M.W., et al. Thiamin, riboflavin and pyridoxine deficiency in psychiatric in-patients. *Br. J. Psychiat.* 141:271–272, 1982.

Christensen, L. The role of caffeine and sugar in depression. *Nutrition Report* 9(3):17–24, March 1991.

Escott-Stump, S. *Nutrition and Diagnosis-Related Care.* Philadelphia: Lea & Febiger, 1988.

Frizel, D., et al. Plasma calcium and magnesium in depression. *Br. J. Psychiat.* 115:1375–1377, 1969.

Ghadirian, A.M., et al. Folic acid deficiency and depression. *Psychosomatics* 21(11):926–929, 1980.

King, D.A. Can allergic exposure provoke psychological symptoms? A double-blind test. *Biol. Psychiat.* 16(1):3–19, 1981.

Leitner, Z.A., et al. Nutritional studies in a mental hospital. *Lancet* 1:215–216, 1975.

Murray, M.; Pizzorno, J. *Encyclopedia of Natural Medicine.* Rocklin, CA: Prima Publishing, 1990.

Shils, M.; Young, V. *Modern Nutrition in Health and Disease.* Philadelphia: Lea & Febiger, 1988.

Stewart, J.W., et al. Low B6 levels in depressed outpatients. *Biol. Psychiat.* 19(4):613–616, 1984.

Diabetes Mellitus

Anderson, J.W.; Ward, K. High-carbohydrate, high-fiber diets for insulin-treated men with diabetes mellitus. *Am. J. Clin. Nutr.* 32:2313–2321, 1979.

Bever, B.O.; Zahand, G.R. Plants with oral hypoglycemic action. *Quart. J. Crude Drug Res.* 17:139–196, 1979.

Escott-Stump, S. *Nutrition and Diagnosis-Related Care.* Philadelpha: Lea & Febiger, 1988.

Kenton, L.; Kenton, S. *Raw Energy.* London: Century Publishing, 1984.

Martinez, O.B., et al. Dietary chromium supplementation on glucose tolerance of elderly Canadian Women. *Nutr. Res.* 5:609–620, 1985.

McCarty, M.F., et al. Rationales for micronutrient supplementation in diabetes. *Med. Hypoth.* 13(2):139–151, 1984.

Murray, M.; Pizzorno, J. *Encyclopedia of Natural Medicine.* Rocklin, CA: Prima Publishing, 1990.

Philipson, H. Dietary fibre in the diabetic diet. *Acta Med. Scand.* (suppl.) 671:91–93, 1983.

Reiser, S., et al. SCOGS report on the health aspects of sucrose consumption. Letter to the Editor. *Am. J. Clinc. Nutr.* 31:9–11, 1978.

Snowdon, D.A.; Phillips, R.L. Does a vegetarian diet reduce the occurrence of diabetes. *Am. J. Public Health* 75(5):507–512, 1985.

Diarrhea

Balch, J.; Balch, P. *Prescription for Nutritional Healing.* Garden City Park, NY: Avery Publishing Group, Inc., 1990.

Carruthers, L.B. Chronic diarrhea treated with folic acid. *Lancet* 1:849, 1946.

Escott-Stump, S. *Nutrition and Diagnosis-Related Care.* Philadelphia: Lea & Febiger, 1988.

Mabey, R. *The New Age Herbalist.* New York: Collier Books, 1988.

Murray, M.; Pizzorno, J. *Encyclopedia of Natural Medicine.* Rocklin, CA: Prima Publishing, 1990.

Diverticulitis

Balch, J.; Balch, P. *Prescription for Nutritional Healing.* Garden City Park, NY: Avery Publishing Group, Inc., 1990.

Krause, M.; Mahan, L. *Food, Nutrition and Diet Therapy.* Philadelphia: W.B.Saunders, 1984.

Eczema

Carper, J. *The Food Pharmacy.* New York: Bantam Books, 1988.

Manku, M.S., et al. Reduced levels of prostaglandin precursors in the blood of atopic patients: defective delta-6 desaturase function as a biochemical basis for atopy. *Prostaglandins Leukotrienes Med.* 9(6):615–638, 1982.

Murray, M.; Pizzorno, J. *Encyclopedia of Natural Medicine.* Rocklin, CA: Prima Publishing, 1990.

Sampson, H.A. Role of immediate food sensitivity in the pathogenesis of atopic dermatitis. *J. Allergy Clin. Immun.* 71:473–480, 1983.

Strosser, A.V., et al. Synthetic vitamin A in the treatment of eczema in children. *Ann. Allergy* 10:703–704, 1952.

Wright, S., et al. Oral evening-primrose-seed oil improves atopic eczema. *Lancet* 1120–1122, November 20, 1982.

Epilepsy and Seizures

Balch, J.; Balch, P. *Prescription for Nutritional Healing.* Garden City Park, NY: Avery Publishing Group, Inc., 1990.

Crayton, J.W., et al. Epilepsy precipitated by food sensitivity: report of a case with double-blind placebo-controlled assessment. *Clin. Electroencephalo.* 12(4)L192–L198, 1981.

Dupont, C.L., et al. Blood manganese levels in children with convulsive disorder. *Biochem. Med.* 33(2):246–255, 1985.

Escott-Stump, S. *Nutrition and Diagnosis-Related Care.* Philadelphia: Lea & Febiger, 1988.

Givverd, F.B., et al. The influence of folic acid on the frequency of epileptic attacks. *Europ. J. Clin. Pharm.* 19(1):57–60, 1981.

Gorges, L.F., et al. Effect of magnesium on epileptic foci. *Epilepsia* 19(1):81–91, 1978.

Krause, M.; Mahan, L. *Food, Nutrition and Diet Therapy.* Philadelphia: W.B.Saunders, 1984.

Lewis-Jones, M.S., et al. Cutaneous manifestions of zinc deficiency during treatment with anticonvulsants. *Brit. Med. J.* 290:604, 1985.

Nakazawa, M. High dose vitamin B_6 therapy in infantile spasms—The effect and adverse reactions. *Brain and Development* 5(2):193, 1983.

Sturman, J. Taurine in nutrition. *Comprehen. Therapy* 3:64, 1977.

Gout

Balch, J.; Balch, P. *Prescription for Nutritional Healing.* Garden City Park, NY: Avery Publishing Group, Inc., 1990.

Blau, L.W. Cherry diet control for gout and arthritis. *Texas Rep. Biol. Med.* 8:309–311, 1950.

Emmerson, B.T. Effect of oral fructose on urate production. *Ann. Rheum. Dis.* 33:276, 1974.

Escott-Stump, S. *Nutrition and Diagnosis-Related Care.* Philadelphia: Lea & Febiger, 1988.

Krause, M.; Mahan, L. *Food, Nutrition and Diet Therapy.* Philadelphia: W.B. Saunders, 1984.

Murray M,; Pizzorno, J. *Encyclopedia of Natural Medicine.* Rocklin, CA: Prima Publishing, 1990.

Shils, M.; Young, V. *Modern Nutrition in Health and Disease.* Philadelphia: Lea & Febiger, 1988.

Stein, H.B., et al. Ascorbic acid-induced uricosuria: a consequence of megavitamin therapy. *Ann. Int. Med.* 84(4):385–388, 1976.

Hair Loss

Balch, J.; Balch, P. *Prescription for Nutritional Healing.* Garden City Park, NY: Avery Publishing Group, Inc., 1990.

Clark, L. *Secrets of Health and Beauty.* New York: Pyramid Books, 1969.

Mabey, R. *The New Age Herbalist.* New York: Collier Books, 1988.

Walker, N.W. *Fresh Vegetable and Fruit Juices.* Prescott, AZ: Norwalk Press, 1970.

Herpes Simplex I and II

Carper, J. *The Food Pharmacy.* New York: Bantam Books, 1988.

Chandra, R.K. Nutrition and immunity—Basic considerations. Part 1. *Contemporary Nutrition* 11(11), 1986.

Griffith, R.; Delong, D.; Nelson, J. Relations of arginine-lysine antagonism to herpes simplex growth in tissue culture. *Chemotherapy* 27:209–213, 1981.

Rhodes, J. Human interferon action: reciprocal regulation by retinoic acid and Beta-carotene. *Journal National Cancer Institute* 70:833–837, 1983.

Terezhalmy, G.T., et al. The use of water soluble bioflavonoid-ascorbic acid complex in the treatment of recurrent herpes labialis. Oral Surgery. Oral Medicine. *Oral Pathology* 45:56–62, 1978.

Hypertension

Douglass, J., et al. Effects of raw food diet on hypertension and obesity. *Southern Medical Journal.* 78(7):841, 1985.

Kaplan, N.M. The non-drug treatment of hypertension. *Ann. Int. Med.* 102:359–373, 1985.

Medeiros, D.M., et al. Blood pressure in young adults as influenced by diet. Anthropometrics, calcium status and serum lipids. *Nutr. Res.* 6:359–368, 1986.

Nonpharmacological approaches to the control of high blood pressure. Final report of the subcommittee on nonpharmacological therapy of the 1984 Joint National Committee Detection, Evaluation, and Treatment of High Blood Pressure. *Hypertension* 8(5):444–467, 1986.

Patki, P.S., et al. Efficiency of potassium and magnesium in essential hypertension: a double blind, placebo controlled, crossover study. *Brit. Med. J.* 301(6751):521–523, 1990.

Smits, P., et al. Circulatory effects of coffee in relation to the pharmacokinetics of caffeine. *American Journal of Cardiology.* 56(15):958–963, 1985.

Hypoglycemia

American Diabetes Association Task Force on Nutrition and Exchange Lists. Nutrition recommendations and principles for individuals with diabetes mellitus. *Diabetes Care* 10:1, 1987.

Anderson, R.A., et al. Chromium supplementation of humans with hypoglycemia. *Fed. Proc.* 43:471, 1984.

Andreani, D.; Mark, V.; Lefebyre, P.J., Eds. *Hypoglycemia.* New York: Raven Press, 1987.

Bells, L.S., et al. Dietary strategies in the treatment of reactive hypoglycemia. *J. Am. Diet. Assoc.* 85:1141, 1985.

Khan, A.; Bryden, N.; et al. Insulin potentiating factor and chromium content of selected foods and spices. *Biological Trace Element Research* 24:183–187, 1990.

Sanders, L.R., et al. Refined carbohydrate as a contributing factor in reactive hypoglycemia. *Southern Medical Journal* 75(9):1072, 1982.

Indigestion

Al-Yahya, M.A.; Rafatullah, S.; et al. Gastroprotective activity of ginger Zingiber Officinale Rosc., in the albino rats. *Am. J. Chinese Med.* 17(1–2):51–56, 1989.

Aroroa, A.; Sharma M.P. Use of banana in non-ulcer dyspepsia. *Lancet* 355: March 1990.

Elta, G.H.; Behler, E.M.; et al. Comparison of coffee intake and coffee-induced symptoms in patients with duodenal ulcer, nonulcer dyspepsia, and normal controls. *American Journal of Gastroenterology* 85(10):1339–1342, 1990.

Hills, B.A.; Kirkwood, C.A. Surfactant approach to the gastric mucosal barrier: protection of rats by banana even when acidified. *Gastroenterology* 97(2):294–303, 1989.

Murray, M.; Pizzorno, J. *Encyclopedia of Natural Medicine.* Rocklin, CA: Prima Publishing, 1990.

Infections

Adetumbi, M.A.; Lau, B.H. Allium sativum (garlic): a natural antibiotic. *Med. Hypoth.* 12(3):227–237, 1983.

Baird, I.M., et al. The effects of ascorbic acid and flavonoids on the occurence of symptoms normally associated with the common cold. *Am. J. Clin. Nutr.* 32:1686–1690, 1979.

Bernstein, J.; Alpert, S.; et al. Depression of lymphocyte transformation following oral glucose ingestion. *Am. J. Clin. Nutr.* 30:613, 1977.

Bondestam, M., et al. Subclinical trace element deficiency in children with an undue susceptibility to infections. *Acta Paediatr. Scandinavia* 74(4):515–520, 1985.

Carper, J. *The Food Pharmacy.* New York: Bantam Books, 1988.

Hussey, G.D.; Klein, M.A. Randomized, controlled trial of vitamin A in children with severe measles. *N. Engl. J. Med.* 323:160–164, 1990.

Shahani, K.M. *Cultured Dairy Products Journal* 12:8–11, 1977.

Inflammation

Al-Yahya, M.A.; Rafatullah, S.; et al. Gastroprotective activity of ginger Zingiber Officinale Rosc., in the albino rats. *Am. J. Chinese Med. 17(1–2):51–56, 1989.*

Amelia, M., et al. Inhibition of mast cell histamine release by flavonoids and bioflavonoids. *Planta Medica* 51:16–20, 1985.

Fletcher, M.; Ziboh, V. Effects of dietary supplementation with eicosapentaenoic acid or gamma-linolenic acid on neutrophil phospholipid fatty acid composition and activation responses. *Inflammation* 14:585–597, 1990.

Skoldstam, L.; Magnusson, K.A. Fasting, intestinal permeability, and rheumatoid arthritis. Rheumatic Disease Clinics of North America. *Nutrition and Rheumatic Diseases* 17(2):363–371, 1991.

Srivastava, K.C.; Mustafa, T. Ginger (Zingiber officinale) and rheumatic disorders. *Med. Hypoth.* 29(1):25–28, 1989.

Taussig, S. The mechanism of the physiological action of bromelain. *Med. Hypoth.* 29(1):25–28, 1989.

Terano, T.; Salmon, J.A.; et al. Eicosapentaenoic acid as a modulator of inflammation effect on prostaglandin and leukotriene synthesis. *Biochemical Pharmacology* 35:799–785, 1986.

Insomnia

Ayers, S.; Mihan, R. Nocturnal leg cramps (systremma): a progress report on response to vitamin E. *Southern Medical Journal* 67(11):1308–1312, 1974.

Boutez, M.I., et al. Neurologic disorders responsive to folic acid therapy. *Can. Med. Assoc. J.* 15:217, 1976.

Growdon, J. Neurotransmitters in the diet; in Wurtman, R.; Wurtman, J., Eds.: *Nutrition and the Brain,* Volume 3. New York: Raven Press, 1979.

Shirlow, M.J.; Mathers, C.D. A study of caffeine consumption and symptoms: indigestion, palpitations, tremor, headache and insomnia. *International Journal of Epidemiology* 14(2):239–248, 1985.

Lyme Disease

Balch, J.; Balch, P. *Prescription for Nutritional Healing.* Garden City Park, NY: Avery Publishing Group, Inc., 1990.

Goodman, S. *Germanium: The Health and Life Enhancer.* Northamptonshire, England: Thorsons Publishing Group, 1988.

Murray, M.; Pizzorno, J. *Encyclopedia of Natural Medicine.* Rocklin, CA: Prima Publishing, 1990.

Memory Loss

Bull, I.R. Vitamin B_{12} and folate status in acute geropsychiatric in-patients. *Nutrition Report* 9(1):1, 1991.

Chernoff, R.; Lipschitz, D.A. Nutrition and aging; in Shils, M.; Young, V.: *Modern Nutrition in Health and Disease.* Philadelphia: Lea & Febinger, 1988.

Moon, C., et al. Main and interaction effects of metallic pollutants on cognitive functioning. *Journal of Learning Disabilities* 18(4):217–221, 1985.

Menopausal Symptoms

British Medical Journal, 905–06, October 20, 1990.

Grist, L.A. *A Woman's Guide to Alternative Medicine.* Ontario, Canada: Beaverbooks, Ltd., 1988.

Kavinoky, N.R. Vitamin E and the control of climacteric symptoms. *Annals Western Med. and Surgery* 4(1):27–32, 1950.

Smith, C.J., et al. Non-hormonal control of vaso-motor flushing in menopausal patients. *Chicago Med.,* March 7, 1964.

Migraine Headache

Egger, J., et al. Is migraine a food allergy: a double-blind controlled trial of olioantigenic diet treatment. *Lancet* ii:865–869, 1983.

Glueck, C.J., et al. Amelioration of severe migraines with omega-3 fatty acids: a double-blind placebo controlled clinical trial. *Am. J. Clin. Nutr.* 43(4):710 (abstract), 1986.

Hanington, E. The platelet and migraine. *Headache* 26:411–415, 1986.

Hughs, E.C., et al. Migraines: a diagnostic test for etiology of food sensitivity by a nutritionally supported fast and confirmed by a long-term report. *Ann. Allergy* 55:28–32, 1985.

Mustafa, T.; Srivastava, K.C. Ginger in migraine headache. *Journal of Ethnopharmacology* 29:267–273, 1990.

Perkins, J.E.; Hartie, J. Diet and migraines: a review of the literature. *J. Am. Diet. Assoc.* 83:459–463, 1983.

Sandler, M., et al. Tyramine sulfoconiugation in relation to depression in migraine. *Journal of Clinical Pain* 5:19–21, 1989.

Motion Sickness

Grontved, A.; Hentzer, E. Vertigo-reducing effect of ginger root. *O.R.L.* 48:282–286, 1986.

Pizzorno, J.; Murray, M. *A Textbook of Natural Medicine.* Seattle: John Bastyr College Publications, 1985.

Wright, J.V. *Dr. Wright's Guide to Healing with Nutrition.* New Canaan, CT: Keats Publishing, 1990.

Muscle Cramps

Ayers, S.; Mihan, R. Nocturnal leg cramps (systremma): a progress report on response to vitamin E. *Southern Medical Journal* 67(11):1308–1312, 1974.

Smith, N.J.; Worthington-Roberts, B. *Food for Sport.* Palo Alto, CA: Bull Publishing Company, 1989.

Osteoporosis

Barger-Lux, M.J., et al. Effects of moderate caffeine intake on the calcium economy of premenopausal women. *Am. J. Clin. Nutr.* 52:722–725, 1990.

Barzel, U.S. Acid loading and osteoporosis. *J. Am. Geriatr. Soc.* 30:613 (letter), 1982.

Dawson-Hughes, B., et al. A controlled trial of the effect of calcium supplementation on bone density in postmenopausal women. *N. Engl. J. Med.* 323:878–883, 1990.

Finkenstedt, G., et al. Lactose absorption, milk consumption, and fasting blood glucose concentrations in women with idiopathic osteoporosis. *Brit. Med. J.* 292:161, 1985.

Goulding, A. Osteoporosis: why consuming less sodium chloride helps conserve bone. *New Zealand Medical Journal* 103:120–122, 1990.

Hollingberry, P.S.; Bergman, E.A.; Massey, L.K. Effect of dietary caffeine and aspirin on urinary calcium and hydroxproline excretion in pre and postmenopausal women. *Fed. Proc.* 44:1149 (abstract #4315), 1985.

Hollingberry, P.S.; Massey, L.K. Effect of dietary caffeine and sucrose on urinary calcium excretion in adolescents. *Fed. Proc.* 45:375 (abstract #1280), 1986.

Jenson, J., et al. Cigarette smoking, serum estrogens, and bone loss during hormone-replacement therapy early after menopause. *N. Engl. J. Med.* 313(16): 973, 1985.

Knapen, M.H.J., et al. The effect of vitamin K supplementation on circulating osteocalcin (bone GLA protein) and urinary calcium excretion. *Ann. Int. Med.* 111:1001–1005, 1989.

Portale, A.A., et al. Oral intake of phosphorus can determine the serum concentrations of 1.25-dihydroxyvitamin D by determining its products rate in humans. *Journal of Clinical Investigations* 77(1): 7, 1986.

Reginister, J.Y., et al. Preliminary report of decreased serum magnesium in postmenopausal osteoporosis. *Magnesium* 8:106–109, 1989.

Zarkadas, M., et al. Sodium chloride supplementation and urinary calcium excretion in postmenopausal women. *Am. J. Clin. Nutr.* 50:1088–1094, 1989.

References

341

Overweight/Obesity

Connor, S.; Connor, W. *The New American Diet.* New York: Fireside, 1986.

Goldbeck, N.; Goldbeck, D. *American Wholefood Cuisine.* New York: New American Library, 1983.

Goldbeck, N.; Goldbeck, D. *The Goldbeck's Guide to Good Food.* New York: New American Library, 1987.

Murray, M.; Pizzorno, J. *Encyclopedia of Natural Medicine.* Rocklin, CA: Prima Publishing, 1990.

Schwartz, Bob. *Diets Don't Work.* Houston: Breakthrough Publishing, 1982.

Periodontal Disease

Alvares, O. Primate studies indicate that subclinical and acute vitamin C deficiency may lead to periodontal disease. *J. A. M. A. 246:730, 1981.*

Carranza, F. *Glickman's Clinical Periodontology.* Philadelphia: W.B. Saunders, 1984.

Kiuchi, F., et al. Inhibitors of prostaglandin biosynthesis from ginger. *Chem. Pharm. Bull. 30:754–757, 1982.*

Ringsdorf, W., et al. Sucrose, neutrophil phagocytosis and resistance to disease. *Dental Survey 52:46–48, 1976.*

Srivastava, K.C.; Mustafa, T. Ginger (Zingiber offinale) and rheumatic disorders. *Med. Hypoth. 29(1):25–28, 1989.*

Taussig, S. The mechanism of the physiological action of bromelain. *Med. Hypoth. 6:99–104, 1980.*

Prostate Enlargement

Bush, I.M., et al. Zinc and the Prostate. Presented at the annual meeting of the American Medical Association, 1974.

Murray, M.; Pizzorno, J. *Encyclopedia of Natural Medicine.* Rocklin, CA: Prima Publishing, 1990.

Wright, J.D. *Dr. Wright's Guide to Healing and Nutrition.* New Canaan, CT: Keats Publishing, 1990.

Psoriasis

Donadini, A., et al. Plasma levels of Zn, Cu, and Ni in healthy controls and psoriatic patients. *Acta Vitaminol. Enzymol. 2:9–16, 1980.*

Lithell, H., et al. A fasting and vegetarian diet treatment trial in chronic inflammatory disorders. *Acta Derm. Vener. Stockholm 63:397–403, 1983.*

Poikolainen, K.; Reunala, T.; et al. Alcohol intake: a risk factor for psoriasis in young and middle-aged men. *Brit. Med. J. 300:780–783, 1990.*

Vahlquist, C., et al. The fatty-acid spectrum in plasma and adipose tissue in patients with psoriasis. *Arch. Dermatol. Res. 278(2): 114–119, 1985.*

Sore Throat

Adetumbi, M.A.; Lau, B.H. Allium sativum (garlic): a natural antibiotic. *Med. Hypoth. 12(3):227–237, 1983.*

Baird, I.M., et al. The effects of ascorbic acid and flavonoids on the occurence of symptoms normally associated with the common cold. *Am. J. Clin. Nutr. 32:1686–1690, 1979.*

Rhodes, J. Human interferon action: reciprocal regulation by retinoic acid and Beta-carotene. *Journal National Cancer Institute 70:833–837, 1983.*

Srivastava, K.C.; Mustafa, T. Ginger (Zingiber officinale) and rheumatic disorders. *Med. Hypoth.* 29(1):25–28, 1989.

Taussig, S. The mechanism of the physiological action of bromelain. *Med. Hypoth.* 6:99–104, 1980.

Surgery Preparation

Gerber, L.E.; Erdman, J.W. Wound healing in rats fed small supplements of retyl acetate, beta-carotene or retinoic acid. *Fed. Proc.*, March 1, 1981.

Kim, J.E.; Shklar, G. The effect of vitamin E on the healing of gingival wounds in rats. *J. Periodontol.* 54:305, 1983.

Olson, R.E. Vitamin K; in Shils, M.; Young, V.: *Modern Nutrition in Health and Disease.* Philadelphia: Lea & Febiger, 1988.

Ringsdorf, W.M.; Cheraskin, E. Vitamin C and human wound healing. *Oral Surg.* 53(3):231–236, 1982.

Srivastava, K.C.; Mustafa, T. Ginger (Zingiber officinale) and rheumatic disorders. *Med. Hypoth.* 29(1):25–28, 1989.

Taussig, S. The mechanism of the physiological action of bromelain. *Med. Hypoth.* 6:99–104, 1980.

Thrombosis

Bordia, A.K. The effect of vitamin C on blood lipids, fibrinolytic activity and platelet adhesiveness in patients with coronary artery disease. *Atherosclerosis* 35:181–187, 1980.

Carper, J. *The Food Pharmacy.* New York: Bantam Books, 1988.

Challen, A.D., et al. The effect of aspirin and linoleic acid on platelet aggregation, platelet fatty acid composition and haemostatis in man.

Hum. Nutr.: Clinc. Nutr. 37(3):197–208, 1983.

Heinicke, R.M., et al. Effect of bromelain (Anase) on human platelet aggregation. *Experientia* 28:844, 1972.

Lam, S.C., et al. Investigation of possible mechanisms of pyridoxal-5-phosphate inhibition of platelet reactions. *Thrombosis Res.* 20:633–645, 1980.

Mitschek, G.H.A. *Experimentelle Pathologie*, Vol.10, 1975.

Renaud, S. Dietary fatty acids and platelet function. *Proc. Nutr. Soc. Aust.* 10:1–13, 1985.

Renaud, S., et al. Protective effects of dietary calcium and magnesium on platelet function and atherosclerosis in rabbits fed saturated fat. *Atherosclerosis* 47:187–198, 1983.

Schone, N.W., et al. Effects of selenium deficiency on aggregation and thromboxane formation in rat platelets. *Fed. Proc.* 43:477, 1984.

Steiner, M., et al. Vitamin E: an inhibitor of the platelet release reaction. *J. Clin. Invest.* 57:732–737, 1976.

Wood, D.A., et al. Linoleic and eicosapentaenoic acids in adipose tissue and platelets and risk of coronary heart disease. *Lancet* 1:176–182, 1987.

Yudkin, J., et al. The relationship between sucrose intake, plasma insulin and platelet adhesiveness in men with and without occlusive vascular disease. *Proc. Nutr. Soc.* 29(1): Suppl:2A–3A, 1970.

Tinnitus

Yanick, P. Nutritional aspects of tinnitus and hearing disorders; in *Tin-*

nitus and Its Management. Yanick, P.; Clark, J.G.: Springfield, IL: Charles C. Thomas, 1984.

Yanick, P.; Gosselin, E.J. Audiologic and metabolic findings in 90 patients with fluctuant hearing loss. *Journal American Audiological Society* 2:15–18, 1975.

Ulcers

Al-Yahya, M.A.; Rafatullah, S.; et al. Gastroprotective activity of ginger Zingiber Officinale Rosc., in the albino rats. *Am. J. Chinese Med.* 17(1–2):51–56, 1989.

Carper, J. *The Food Pharmacy*. New York: Bantam Books, 1988.

Cheney, G. Anti-peptic ulcer dietary factor. *J. Am. Diet. Assoc.* 26:668–672, 1950.

Elta, G.H.; Behler, E.M.; et al. Comparison of coffee intake and coffee-induced symptoms in patients with duodenal ulcer, nonulcer dyspepsia, and normal controls. *Am. J. Gastroenterology* 85(10): 1339–1342, 1990.

Hills, B.A.; Kirkwood, C.A. Surfactant approach to the gastric mucosal barrier: protection of rats by banana even when acidified. *Gastroenterology* 97(2):294–303, 1989.

Katschinski, B.D., et al. Duodenal ulcer and refined carbohydrate intake: a case-control study assessing dietary fibre and refined sugar intake. *Gut* 31(9):993–996, 1990.

Russel, R.L., et al. Ascorbic acid levels in leucocytes of patients with gastrointestinal hemorrhage. *Lancet* 2:603–606, 1968.

Underweight

Souba, W.W.; Wilmore, D.W. Diet and nutrition in the care of patients with surgery, trauma, and sepsis; in Shils, M.; Young, V.: *Modern Nutrition in Health and Disease*. Philadelphia: Lea & Febiger, 1988.

Varicose Veins

Gabor, M. The pharmacologic effects of flavonoids on blood vessels. *Angiologica* 9:355–374, 1972.

Rose, S. What causes varicose veins. *Lancet* i:32, 1986.

Taussig, S. The mechanism of the physiological action of bromelain. *Med. Hypoth.* 6:99–104, 1980.

Water Retention

Murray, M.; Pizzorno, J. *Encyclopedia of Natural Medicine*. Rocklin, CA: Prima Publishing, 1990.

Roe, D. Diet, nutrition, and drug reactions; in Shils, M.; Young, V.: *Modern Nutrition in Health and Disease*. Philadelphia: Lea & Febiger, 1988.

Strinivasan, S.R., et al. Effects of dietary sodium and sucrose on the induction of hypertension in spider monkeys. *Am. J. Clin. Nutr.*, 561–569, March 1980.

Index

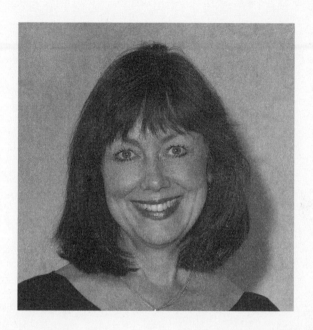

CHERIE CALBOM, M.S., is the author of fifteen books, including *The Wrinkle Cleanse* and *The Juice Lady's Guide to Juicing for Health*, as well as the best-selling *George Foreman's Knock-Out-the-Fat Barbecue and Grilling Cookbook*, *The Ultimate Smoothie Book*, and *The Coconut Diet*. She earned a master of science degree in nutrition from Bastyr University, where she now sits on the Board of Regents. She has appeared on QVC regularly for more than ten years with the George Foreman grills and the Juiceman juicer. Calbom is known as "The Juice Lady" for her work with juicing and health, and her juice therapy and cleansing programs have been popular for more than a decade. For more on her books and programs, see http://www.juicinginfo.net.

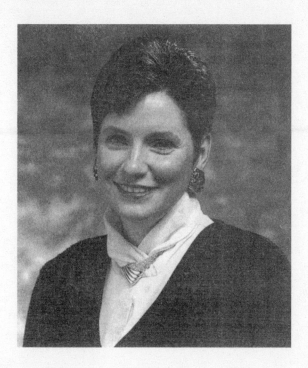

MAUREEN KEANE, M.S., C.N., is a Washington State certified nutritionist and member of the American Dietetic Association. She received her undergraduate degree in biology from Wayne State University in Michigan and her master's degree in nutrition from Bastyr University in Washington State. Maureen is the best-selling author of more than thirteen books on health and nutrition, and her articles appear on Internet health sites such as WebMD. Her two books on cancer nutrition are recommended by most cancer treatment centers in the United States.

Maureen is a cancer treatment survivor herself; chemotherapy and surgery left her with both fibromyalgia and hidden damage to her lungs. The latter led to heart failure and a ten-year battle to regain her health. She is convinced a whole-foods diet rich in fruits and vegetables and their juices could have protected her healthy cells from the friendly fire of cancer treatment and prevented this damage. If you have questions about juicing, weight loss, or nutrition, Maureen invites you to her website for more information: www.keanenutrition.com.

Also available from Cherie Calbom, M.S.

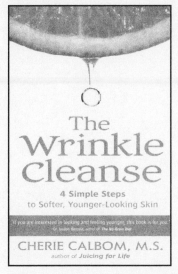

The Wrinkle Cleanse: 4 Simple Steps
to Softer, Younger-Looking Skin

ISBN 1-58333-255-3; 978-1-58333-255-9

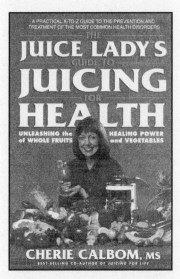

The Juice Lady's Guide to Juicing for Health:
Unleashing the Healing Power of Whole Fruits and Vegetables

ISBN 0-89529-999-2; 978-0-89529-999-4